1

By the Author of

Epilepsy You're Not Alone

Breast Cancer: Questions,
Answers & Self-Help
Techniques

Author

STACEY CHILLEMI

Breast Cancer: Questions, Answers & Self-Help Techniques

2007 Author Stacey Chillemi

For more information regarding permission, email to:
Author Stacey Chillemi
staceychil@aol.com
Designed and produced by Stacey Chillemi
ISBN: 978-1-4357-2137-1
Printed in the U.S.A.

Special Edition, April 2007

ACKNOWLEDGMENTS

I feel blessed that I have family and friends who are as wonderful as my friends are. My family and friends stood by my side, helped me, and supported me with their love encouragement and prayers. I especially want to thank my wonderful husband, Michael, for his love and sacrifice, and my three children, Mikey, Alexis, and Anthony, who opened my eyes to see the beauty of life in a completely different light. They made me realize how precious life is and they give me the motivation and reason to live a positive lifestyle and to do everything I can to make sure I am healthy and fit.

I am also extremely grateful to Marie, my best friend, who has been there for me since we were kids. I would also like to convey my love and appreciation to my friend Michelle who is a breast cancer survivor and Terri Gill who is like family. Terri and Michelle were my motivation for writing this book. I have never seen so much strength in these two people. The stories they shared, their positive attitudes, their displays of strength were unbelievable.

Michelle and Terri never gave up and with the support of their family and friends; both of them fought breast cancer and came out of the battle a winner and a true hero. This book is for you Terri and Michelle.

FORWARD

All my life I have been writing books and poetry about epilepsy. As I have been getting older now in my mid-thirties I have seen several of my friends develop breast cancer and other types of cancers.

I have learned over the years that words can be very powerful and can change a person's life. I myself have not experienced breast cancer, but I wrote this book to help educate women about breast cancer, so they can help prevent it or catch it in the early stages when it can be treated and cured. I also wanted to teach my coping skills and techniques. These powerful techniques were created to help women with breast cancer.

Today, approximately one in almost every eight women (13.4%) will develop breast cancer in her lifetime. Why take changes with your life. I have learned over the years that doctors are people too, not miracle workers. It is up to us to research and do what ever possible to help maintain a happy, healthy and productive life.

CONTENTS

9

1. What Is Breast Cancer?

Each month, a woman's breasts go through temporary changes associated with menstruation, and a lump may form. While the vast majority of these growths are not cancerous, any lump should be examined immediately.

Lumps are most common in the lobules -- small sacs that produce milk -- or the ducts that carry milk to the nipple. But they occasionally start in other tissue. The two main categories of breast cancer are lobular and ductal carcinomas.

Anatomy of the Breast

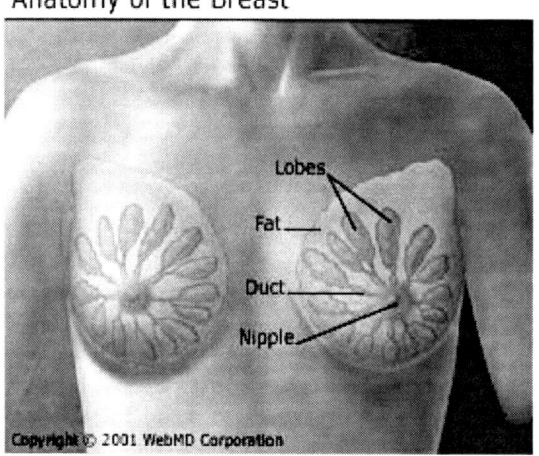

Copyright © 2001 WebMD Corporation

Breast cancer usually begins with the formation of a small, confined tumor. Some tumors are benign, meaning they do not invade other tissue; others are malignant, or cancerous. Malignant tumors have the potential to metastasize, or spread. Once such a tumor grows to a certain size, it is more likely to shed cells that spread to other parts of the body through the bloodstream and lymphatic system. Different types of breast cancer grow and spread at different rates; some take years to spread beyond the breast, while others move quickly.

Men can get breast cancer, too, but they account for less than one-half of one percent of all cases. Among women, breast cancer is the most common cancer and the second leading cause of cancer deaths -- behind lung cancer.

If eight women were to live to be at least 85, one of them would be expected to develop the disease at some point during her life. Two-thirds of women with breast cancer are over 50, and most of the rest are between 39 and 49.

Fortunately, breast cancer is very treatable if detected early. Localized tumors can usually be treated successfully before the cancer spreads; and in nine in 10 cases, the woman will live at least another five years. Experts usually consider a five-year survival to be a cure.

Once the cancer begins to spread, getting rid of it completely is more difficult, although treatment can often control the disease for years. Improved screening procedures and treatment options mean that at least seven out of 10 women with breast cancer will survive more than five years after initial diagnosis, and half will survive more than 10 years.

What Causes Breast Cancer?

Although the precise causes of breast cancer are unclear, we know what the main risk factors are. Still, most women considered at high risk for breast cancer do not get it, while many who do have no known risk factors. Among the most significant factors are advancing age and a family history of breast cancer. Risk increases slightly for a woman who has had a benign breast lump and increases significantly for a woman who has previously had cancer of the breast or the ovaries.

A woman whose mother, sister, or daughter has had breast cancer is two to three times more likely to develop the disease, particularly if more than one first-degree relative has been affected. Researchers have now identified two genes responsible for some instances of familial breast cancer -- called *BRCA1* and *BRCA2*. About one woman in 200 carries it. Having the gene predisposes a woman to breast cancer but does not ensure that she will get it.

Generally, women over 50 are more likely to get breast cancer than younger women, and African-American women are more likely than Caucasions to get breast cancer before menopause.

A link between breast cancer and hormones is gradually becoming clearer. Researchers think that the greater a woman's exposure to the hormone estrogen, the more susceptible she is to breast cancer. Estrogen tells cells to divide; the more the cells divide, the more likely they are to be abnormal in some way, possibly becoming cancerous.

A woman's exposure to estrogen and progesterone rises and falls during her lifetime, influenced by the age she starts and stops menstruating, the average length of her menstrual cycle, and her age at first childbirth. A woman's risk for breast cancer is increased if she starts menstruating before age 12, has her first child after 30, stops menstruating after 55, or has a menstrual cycle shorter or longer than the average 26-29 days. Current information indicates that the hormones in birth control pills probably do not increase the risk. Some studies suggest that taking hormone replacement therapy after menopause may increase risk, especially when taken for more than 5 years. The jury is still somewhat out on this matter though. Heavy doses of radiation therapy may also be a factor, but low-dose mammograms pose almost no risk.

The link between diet and breast cancer is debated. Obesity is a noteworthy risk factor, and drinking alcohol regularly -- more than a couple of drinks a day -- may promote the disease. Many studies have shown that women whose diets are high in fat are more likely to get the disease. Researchers suspect that if a woman lowers her daily calories from fat -- to less than 20%-30% -- her diet may help protect her from developing breast cancer.

2. How Does Breast Cancer Begin?

Breast cancer is the most common cancer among women, after nonmelanoma skin cancer. Over the past 50 years, the number of women diagnosed with the disease has increased each year. Today, approximately one in almost every eight women (13.4%) will develop breast cancer in her lifetime. Breast cancer is the second-leading cause of cancer death in women after lung cancer -- and is the leading cause of cancer death among women ages 35 to 54. The American Cancer Society estimates that approximately 211,240 women are going to be diagnosed with invasive breast cancer and approximately 40,410 will die. Although these numbers may sound frightening, research reveals that the mortality rate could decrease by 30% if all women age 50 and older who need a mammogram had one.

As a woman, I firmly believe that we cannot wait until the doctors diagnose us with a frightening disease, such as breast cancer and hope for a miracle cure. It is up to each individual to educate themselves, understand what breast cancer is, how it is caused and how we can help ourselves, so the chances of getting breast cancer is increasing low.

How does breast cancer begin?

First, I would like to explain to you how breast cancer begins. The cells in our breasts normally reproduce only when new cells are needed. Sometimes, cells in a part of the body grow and reproduce out of control, which creates a mass of tissue called a tumor. If the cells that are growing out of control are normal cells, the tumor is called benign which means not cancerous. If however, the cells that are growing out of control are abnormal and they do not function like the body's normal cells, the tumor is called malignant which means the tumor is cancerous.

Cancers are named after the part of the body from which they originate. Breast cancer originates in the breast tissue. Like other cancers, breast cancer can infect and grow into the tissue surrounding the breast. It can also travel to other parts of the body and form new tumors, a process called metastasis.

The medical field is still unsure what causes breast cancer; they do know that certain risk factors may put you at higher risk of developing it. A person's age, genetic factors, personal health history and diet all contribute to breast cancer.

3. What Causes Breast Cancer?

Although the precise causes of breast cancer are unclear, we know what the main risk factors are. Still, most women considered at high risk for breast cancer do not get it, while many who do have no known risk factors. Among the most significant factors are advancing age and a family history of breast cancer. Risk increases slightly for a woman who has had a benign breast lump and increases significantly for a woman who has previously had cancer of the breast or the ovaries.

A woman whose mother, sister, or daughter has had breast cancer is two to three times more likely to develop the disease, particularly if more than one first-degree relative has been affected. Researchers have now identified two genes responsible for some instances of familial breast cancer -- called *BRCA1* and *BRCA2*. About one woman in 200 carries it. Having the gene predisposes a woman to breast cancer but does not ensure that she will get it.

Generally, women over 50 are more likely to get breast cancer than younger women, and African-American women are more likely than Caucasions to get breast cancer before menopause.

A link between breast cancer and hormones is gradually becoming clearer. Researchers think that the greater a woman's exposure to the hormone estrogen, the more susceptible she is to breast cancer. Estrogen tells cells to divide; the more the cells divide, the more likely they are to be abnormal in some way, possibly becoming cancerous.

A woman's exposure to estrogen and progesterone rises and falls during her lifetime, influenced by the age she starts and stops menstruating, the average length of her menstrual cycle, and her age at first childbirth. A woman's risk for breast cancer is increased if she starts menstruating before age 12, has her first child after 30, stops menstruating after 55, or has a menstrual cycle shorter or longer than the average 26-29 days. Current information indicates that the hormones in birth control pills probably do not increase the risk. Some studies suggest that taking hormone replacement therapy after

16

menopause may increase risk, especially when taken for more than 5 years. The jury is still somewhat out on this matter though. Heavy doses of radiation therapy may also be a factor, but low-dose mammograms pose almost no risk.

The link between diet and breast cancer is debated. Obesity is a noteworthy risk factor, and drinking alcohol regularly -- more than a couple of drinks a day -- may promote the disease. Many studies have shown that women whose diets are high in fat are more likely to get the disease. Researchers suspect that if a woman lowers her daily calories from fat -- to less than 20%-30% -- her diet may help protect her from developing breast cancer.

4. The Risk Factors of Breast Cancer

Every woman is at SOME risk for breast cancer—this is merely the "risk" of living as a woman. However, many risk factors can make one woman's picture differ substantially from another's. When you understand your own particular risk profile, you are in a better position to manage it and do not have to fear the unknown.

Reasonably higher risk

- **Getting older**. Your risk for breast cancer increases as you age. About 77% of women diagnosed with breast cancer each year are over age 50, and almost half are age 65 and older. Consider this: In women 40 to 49 years of age, there is a one in 68 - risk of developing breast cancer. In the 50 to 59 age group, that risk increases to one in 37.

- **Direct family history**. Having a mother, sister or daughter ("first degree" relative) who has breast cancer puts you at higher risk for the disease. The risk is even greater if your relative developed breast cancer before menopause and had cancer in both breasts. Having one first-degree relative with breast cancer approximately doubles a woman's risk, and having two first-degree relatives increases her risk 5-fold. Having a male blood relative with breast cancer will also increase a woman's risk of the disease.

- **Genetics**. Carriers of alterations in either of two familial breast cancer genes called BRCA1 or BRCA2 are at higher risk. Women with an inherited alteration in either of these genes have up to an 80% chance of developing breast cancer in their lifetime.

- **Breast lesions**. A previous breast biopsy result of atypical hyperplasia (lobular or ductal) increases a woman's breast cancer risk by four to five times.

Somewhat higher risk

- **Distant family history**. This refers to breast cancer in more distant relatives such as aunts, grandmothers and cousins.

- **Previous abnormal breast biopsy**. Women with earlier biopsies showing any of the following have a slight increased risk: fibroadenomas with complex features, hyperplasia without atypia, sclerosing adenosis and solitary papilloma.

- **Age at childbirth**. Having your first child after age 30 or never having children puts you at higher risk.

- **Early menstruation**. Your risk increases if you got your period before age 12.
- **Late menopause**. If you begin menopause after age 55, your risk increases.

- **Weight**. Being overweight (especially in the waist), with excess caloric and fat intake, increases your risk, especially after menopause.

- **Excessive radiation**. This is especially true for women who were given radiation for postpartum mastitis, received prolonged fluoroscopic X-rays for tuberculosis or who were exposed to a large amount of radiation before age 30 -- usually as treatment for cancers such as lymphoma.

- **Other cancer in the family**. A family history of cancer of the ovaries, cervix, uterus or colon increases your risk.

- **Heritage**. Female descendents of Eastern and Central European Jews (Ashkenazi) are at increased risk.

- **Alcohol**. Use of alcohol is linked to increased risk of developing breast cancer. Compared with nondrinkers, women who consume one alcoholic drink a day have a very small increase in risk, and those who have 2 to 5 drinks daily, have about 1.5 times the risk of women who drink no alcohol.

Alcohol is also known to increase the risk of developing cancers of the mouth, throat, and esophagus.

- **Race**. Caucasian women are at a slightly higher risk of developing breast cancer than are African-American, Asian, Hispanic and Native American women.

- **Hormone Replacement Therapy (HRT)**. Long-term use of combined estrogen and progesterone increases the risk of breast cancer. This risk seems to return to that of the general population after discontinuing them for 5 years or more.

Low risk

- Pregnancy before age 18.
- Early onset of menopause.
- Surgical removal of the ovaries before age 37.

Factors not related to breast cancer

- Abortion or miscarriage.
- Fibrocystic breast changes.
- Multiple pregnancies.
- Coffee or caffeine intake.
- Antiperspirants.
- Under wire bras.
- Breast implants.

Only 5-10% of breast cancers occur in women who developed cancer because it is in their family heritage. Most women who get cancer have no direct family history of the disease. The risk for developing breast cancer increases as a woman gets older.

5. The Warning Signs

The warning signs of breast cancer include:

1. Lump or thickening in, near the breast, or in the underarm that persists through the menstrual cycle.
2. A mass or lump, which may feel as small as a pea.
3. A change in the size, shape or contour of the breast.
4. A bloodstained or clear fluid discharge from the nipple.
5. A change in the feel or appearance of the skin on the breast or nipple (dimpled, puckered, scaly or inflamed).
6. Redness of the skin on the breast or nipple.
7. An area that is distinctly different from any other area on either breast.
8. A marble-like hardened area under the skin.

These changes may be found when performing monthly breast self-exams. By performing breast self-exams, you can become familiar with the normal monthly changes in your breasts.

6. How to Perform a Breast Self-Exam

Breast self-examination should be performed at the same time each month, three to five days after your menstrual period ends. If you have stopped menstruating, perform the exam on the same day of each month.

How to Perform a Breast Self-Exam:

In the mirror:

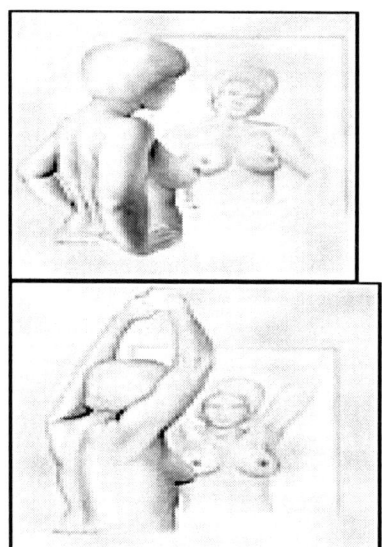

1. Stand undressed from the waist up in front of a large mirror in a well-lit room. Look at your breasts. Do not be alarmed if they do not look equal in size or shape. Most women's breasts are not. With your arms relaxed by your sides, look for any changes in size, shape or position, or any changes to the skin of the breasts. Look for any skin puckering, dimpling, sores or discoloration. Inspect your nipples and look for

any sores, peeling or change in the direction of the nipples.

2. Next, place your hands on your hips and press down firmly to tighten the chest muscles beneath your breasts. Turn from side to side so you can inspect the outer part of your breasts.

3. Then bend forward toward the mirror. Roll your shoulders and elbows forward to tighten your chest muscles. Your breasts will fall forward. Look for any changes in the shape or contour of your breasts.

4. Now, clasp your hands behind your head and press your hands forward. Again, turn from side to side to inspect your breasts' outer portions. Remember to inspect the border underneath your breasts. You may need to lift your breasts with your hand to see this area.

5. Check your nipples for discharge (fluid). Place your thumb and forefinger on the tissue surrounding the nipple and pull outward toward the end of the nipple. Look for any discharge. Repeat on your other breast.

In the shower

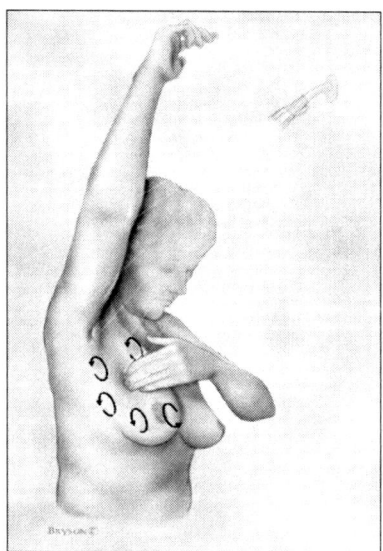

6. Now, it is time to feel for changes in the breast. It is helpful to have your hands slippery with soap and water. Check for any lumps or thickening in your underarm area. Place your left hand on your hip and reach with your right hand to feel in the left armpit. Repeat on the other side.

7. Check both sides for lumps or thickenings above and below your collarbone.

8. With hands soapy, raise one arm behind your head to spread out the breast tissue. Use the flat part of your fingers from the other hand to press gently into the breast. Follow an up-and-down pattern along the breast, moving from bra line to collarbone. Continue the pattern until you have covered the entire breast. Repeat on the other side.

Lying down

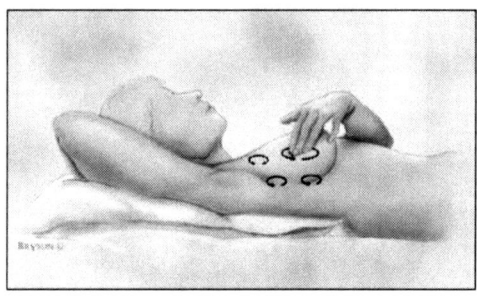

9. Next, lie down and place a small pillow or folded towel under your right shoulder. Put your right hand behind your head. Place your left hand on the upper portion of your right breast with fingers together and flat. Body lotion may help to make this part of the exam easier.

10. Think of your breast as a face on a clock. Start at 12 o'clock and move toward 1 o'clock in small circular motions. Continue around the entire circle until you reach 12 o'clock again. Keep your fingers flat and in constant contact with your breast. When the circle is complete, move in one inch toward the nipple and complete another circle around the clock. Continue in this pattern until you have felt the entire breast. Make sure to feel the upper outer areas that extend into your armpit.

11. Place your fingers flat and directly on top of your nipple. Feel beneath the nipple for any changes. Gently press your nipple inward. It should move easily.

Repeat steps 9, 10 and 11 on your other breast.

Cancerous tumors are more likely to be found in certain parts of the breast over others. If you divide the breast into 4 sections, the approximate percentage of breast cancers found in each area are (in clockwise pattern):

- 41% upper, outer quadrant
- 14% upper, inner quadrant
- 5% lower, inner quadrant
- 6% lower, outer quadrant
- 34% in the area behind the nipple

Almost half occur in the upper outer quadrant of the breast, towards the armpit. Some physicians refer to this region as the "tail" of the breast and encourage women to examine it closely.

If you detect a lump, go immediately to your doctor. Changes in your breast that should be checked by your doctor **include:**

- An area that is distinctly different from any other area on either breast.

- A lump or thickening in, near the breast, or in the underarm that persists through the menstrual cycle.

- A change in the size, shape or contour of the breast.

- A mass or lump, which may feel as small as a pea.

- A marble-like area under the skin.

- A change in the feel or appearance of the skin on the breast or nipple (dimpled, puckered, scaly or inflamed).

- Bloody or clear fluid discharge from the nipples.

- Redness of the skin on the breast or nipple.

- **Invasive ductal carcinoma**. This cancer starts in the milk ducts of the breast. Then it breaks through the wall of the duct and invades the fatty tissue of the breast. This is the most common form of breast cancer, accounting for 80% of invasive cases.

- **Ductal carcinoma in situ (DCIS)** is ductal carcinoma in its earliest stage (stage 0). In situ refers to the fact that the cancer has not spread beyond its point of origin. In this case, the disease is confined to the milk ducts and it has not invaded nearby breast tissue. If untreated, ductal carcinoma in situ may become invasive cancer. It is usually curable.

- **Infiltrating (invasive) lobular carcinoma**. This cancer begins in the lobules of the breast where breast milk is produced, but has spread to surrounding tissues or the rest of the body. It accounts for about 10% of invasive breast cancers.

- **Lobular carcinoma in situ (LCIS)** is cancer that is only in the lobules of the breast. It is not a true cancer, but serves as a marker for the increased risk of developing breast cancer later, possibly in both breasts. This is why it is important for women with lobular carcinoma in situ to have regular clinical breast exams and mammograms.

7. The Stages of Breast Cancer

- Early stage or stage 0 breast cancer is when the disease is localized to the breast with no evidence of spread to the lymph nodes (carcinoma in situ).

- Stage 1 breast cancer: The cancer is two centimeters or less in size and it has not spread anywhere.

- Stage 2A breast cancer is a tumor smaller than two centimeters across with lymph node involvement or a tumor that is larger than two are but less than five centimeters across without underarm lymph node involvement.

- Stage 2B is a tumor that is greater than five centimeters across without underarm lymph nodes testing positive for cancer or a tumor that is larger than two but less than five centimeters across with lymph node involvement.

- Advanced breast cancer (metastatic) results after cancer cells spread to the lymph nodes and to other parts of the body.

- Another name for stage 3A breast cancer is called locally advanced breast cancer. The tumor is larger than five centimeters and has spread to the lymph nodes under the arm, or a tumor that is any size with cancerous lymph nodes that adhere to one another or surrounding tissue.

- Stage 3B breast cancer is a tumor of any size that has spread to the skin, chest wall or internal mammary lymph nodes (located beneath the breast and inside the chest).

- Stage 3C breast cancer is a tumor of any size that has spread more extensively and involves more lymph node invasion.

- Stage 4-breast cancer is defined as a tumor, regardless of size, that has spread to places far away from the breast, such as bones, lungs, liver, brain or distant lymph nodes.

8. How is Breast Cancer Diagnosed?

During your regular physical examination, your doctor will take a careful personal and family history and perform a breast exam and possibly one or more other tests:

- Mammography
- Ultrasonography

Based on the results of these tests, your doctor may or may not request a biopsy to get a sample of the breast mass cells or tissue.

After the sample is removed, it is sent to a lab for testing. A pathologist -- a doctor who specializes in diagnosing abnormal tissue changes -- views the sample under a microscope and looks for abnormal cell shapes or growth patterns. When cancer is present, the pathologist can tell what kind of cancer it is (ductal or lobular carcinoma) and whether it has spread beyond the ducts or lobules.

Laboratory tests such as hormone receptor tests (estrogen and progesterone) can show whether the hormones help the cancer to grow. If the test results show that hormones help the cancer grow (a positive test), the cancer is likely to respond to hormonal treatment. This therapy deprives the cancer of the estrogen hormone.

A team of experts working together with the patient best accomplishes breast cancer diagnosis and treatment. Each patient needs to evaluate the advantages and limitations of each type of treatment, and work with her team of physicians to develop the best approach.

9. How is Breast Cancer Treated?

If the tests find cancer, you and your doctor will develop a treatment plan to eradicate the breast cancer, to reduce the chance of cancer returning in the breast, as well as to reduce the chance of the cancer traveling to a location outside of the breast. Treatment generally follows within a few weeks after the diagnosis.

The type of treatment recommended will depend on the size and location of the tumor in the breast, the results of lab tests done on the cancer cells and the stage or extent of the disease. Your doctor usually considers your age and general health as well as your feelings about the treatment options.

Breast cancer treatments are local or systemic.

- Local treatments are used to remove, destroy or control the cancer cells in a specific area, such as the breast. Surgery and radiation treatment are local treatments.

- Systemic treatments are used to destroy or control cancer cells all over the body. Chemotherapy and hormone therapy such as tamoxifen, and biologic therapies like Herceptin, are systemic treatments. A patient may have just one form of treatment or a combination, depending on her needs.

10. What Happens After Treatment?

Following local breast cancer treatment, the treatment team will determine the chances that the cancer will recur outside the breast. This team usually includes a medical oncologist, who is a specialist trained in using medicines to treat breast cancer. The medical oncologist, who works with the surgeon, may advise the use of tamoxifen or possibly chemotherapy. These treatments are used in addition to, but not in place of, local breast cancer treatment with surgery and/or radiation therapy.

How You Can Protect Yourself from Breast Cancer

Follow these three steps for early detection:

1. Get a mammogram. The American Cancer Society recommends having a baseline mammogram at age 35 and a screening mammogram every year after age 40. Mammograms are an important part of your health history. If you go to another healthcare provider, or move, take the film (mammogram) with you.

2. Examine your breasts each month after age 20. You will become familiar with the contours and feel of your breasts and will be more alert to changes.

3. Have your breast examined by a healthcare provider at least once every three years after age 20, and every year after age 40. Clinical breast exams can detect lumps that may not be detected by mammogram.

Section 2

Recovery

11. Nutrition

Nutrition—giving your body the nutrients it needs—is important for everyone. When combined with exercising and maintaining a healthy weight, eating well is an excellent way to keep your body healthy.

If you have a personal history of breast cancer or are at high risk for the disease, eating well is particularly important for you. In this section, you can read about healthy eating, how nutrition may help reduce your risk of a first-time breast cancer or breast cancer recurrence, and what and how to eat during and after treatment.

Healthy eating means eating a variety of foods that give you the nutrients you need to maintain your health, feel good, and have energy. These nutrients include protein, carbohydrates, fat, water, vitamins, and minerals.

Nutrition is important for everyone. When combined with being physically active and maintaining a healthy weight, eating well is an excellent way to help your body stay strong and healthy. If you have a history of breast cancer or are at high risk for the disease, eating well is especially important for you. What you eat can affect your immune system, your mood, and your energy level.

12. Understanding Food Groups

Fruits and Vegetables

Cancer experts as well as registered dietitians recommend a diet rich in fruits and vegetables. The American Cancer Society and the American Institute for Cancer Research recommend eating five or more servings of a variety of vegetables and fruits each day to ensure that your cancer risk is as low as it can be. The U.S. Department of Agriculture (USDA) 2005 Dietary Guidelines for Americans recommend nine servings of fruit and vegetables each day. This sounds like a lot, but it is really only about 2 cups of fruit and two and a half cups of vegetables.

Nutrition experts say that variety is key, because different fruits and vegetables have different nutrients. Also, if you eat too much of one thing, you will get bored. One way to eat a variety of fruits and vegetables is to eat foods with all the colors of the rainbow. Green is broccoli. Red is peppers. Yellow is a banana. Purple is eggplant. Orange is an orange. Alternatively, try to eat dark green vegetables (think spinach, collard greens, or kale) at one meal, and orange (carrots, sweet potatoes, or squash) the next. Cut up an apple into your morning cereal and have a peach with your lunch. Frozen raspberries or blackberries are a yummy dessert. Be creative!

Whole Grains

USDA guidelines recommend three ounces or more of whole grains per day. Whole grains still have the bran and the germs (the core of the grain kernel) attached and have more fiber, minerals, and vitamins than refined grains. The refining process removes the bran and germ from the grain.

You cannot tell if a food is produced from whole grain by looking at its color—you have to read the label. The ingredients should say "whole" or "whole grain" before the grain's name, "whole grain wheat," for example. Brown rice, bulgur, oatmeal, and barley are other examples of whole grains that are eaten on their own. Both the American Institute for Cancer Research and the American Cancer Society recommend choosing whole grains over refined grains. In order, to be considered high in whole grains, bread must have two to three grams of fiber per slice, and cereals must have at least six or more grams of fiber per serving. Some examples are Multi-Bran Chex cereal by General Mills (seven grams of fiber per serving) and Flax and Fiber Crunch cereal by Back to Nature (nine grams of fiber per serving).

Meat and Beans

Meat is a good source of the protein and fatty acids you need for energy and health. Red meat also contains iron, which is especially important for women. However, meat also has high levels of saturated fat and cholesterol. The USDA guidelines recommend five and a half ounces of meat (defined to include chicken and fish) per day, or meat substitutes (vegetable protein products) or beans if you prefer not to eat meat. If you do eat meat, poultry, or fish, try to choose lean cuts and opt for chicken or fish most of the time. If you do not eat meat, you may need to add nuts, seeds, or dry beans to your diet to ensure that you are getting enough protein and iron.

Eggs are also included in this category. One egg equals a one-ounce serving of meat.

Milk/Dairy

The USDA recommends that you eat, every day,

- Three cups of low-fat/fat-free milk or yogurt (that's a little more than three six-ounce containers of yogurt), or

- Four and a half ounces of low-fat/fat-free natural cheese, such as cheddar (about 4 slices), or

- Six ounces of low fat or fat-free processed cheese, such as American (about six slices).

Processed cheese has less calcium than natural cheese. That is why you need to eat more of it per day. Processed cheese is made from natural cheese and other ingredients. It is pasteurized and has more moisture so it can be stored longer and melts easier.

Eating these recommended amounts of dairy foods each day will give you the amount of calcium you need.

If you do not like or cannot drink milk or milk products, make sure you get enough phosphorus, vitamin A, calcium, and vitamin D from other food sources. If you are lactose intolerant, you might want to try lactase supplements.

Oils

Butter, canola oil, olive oil—you need some of these, but not very much. The USDA guidelines recommend two to three teaspoons of these high-calorie but oh-so-tasty flavorings per day.

Oils are fats. **There are three main types of fats.**

Saturated fats are the "bad" fats that raise your cholesterol levels. These fats include trans fat, found in shortening, stick (or hard) margarine, cookies, crackers, snack foods, fried foods, doughnuts, pastries, baked goods, and other processed foods made with or fried in partially hydrogenated oils.

Monounsaturated fat and polyunsaturated fats are the "good" fats that help lower your LDL cholesterol.

These five food groups can supply you with all the nutrients your body needs to stay healthy and strong. You may be wondering where chocolate and some of your other favorite treats fit. Do not worry, they do. You just have to think about when you eat them and how much of them you eat. First, let us look at how your body uses the foods you eat.

13. Getting Nutrients from Foods

Eating a wide range of foods that include a variety of nutrients is the easiest way to have a healthy diet.

- Proteins give your body amino acids—the building blocks that help your body's cells do all of their everyday activities. Proteins help your body build new cells, repair old cells, create hormones and enzymes, and keep your immune system healthy. If you do not, have enough protein, your body takes longer to recover from illness, and you are more likely to get sick. During treatment for breast cancer, women may need more protein than usual.

- Carbohydrates give your body a little more than half of the calories it needs to function each day. Carbohydrates give you quick energy—which is why you hear about athletes "carbo loading" before a big event. They are fueling their bodies for the challenge to come.

- Fruits, vegetables, bread, pasta, grains, cereal products, crackers, dried beans, peas, and lentils are all good sources of carbohydrates. Many of them are also good sources of fiber, which your digestive system needs to, stay healthy. Sugar (white and brown), honey, and molasses are also carbohydrates. However, these types of carbohydrates are high in calories and do not offer any other benefits (like vitamins and minerals). Whole grains, fruits and vegetables are healthier sources of carbs than refined grains and sugars.

- Fats give your body the fatty acids it needs to grow and to produce new cells and hormones. Fat also helps some vitamins move through your body. Vitamins A, D, E, and K are fat-soluble vitamins, which means they need some fat to be absorbed. They are also stored in the fatty tissues in your body and the liver. Fat also helps protect your organs against trauma. Your body stores excess calories as fat, which is saved up as reserve energy.

There are three basic types of fats:

- Saturated fats, found mainly in meat and whole milk products, are only found in foods that come from animals, not those that come from plants. Saturated fat is the type that raises your blood cholesterol level. Trans fats (also called trans-saturated fats or trans fatty acids) are formed when liquid vegetable oils go through a process called hydrogenation, in which hydrogen is added to make the oils more solid. Hydrogenated vegetable fats are used in food processing because they give foods a longer shelf life and a desirable taste, shape, and texture. The majority of trans fat is found in shortening, stick (or hard) margarine, cookies, crackers, snack foods, fried foods (including fried fast food), doughnuts, pastries, baked goods, and other processed foods made with or fried in partially hydrogenated oils. Trans fat also raises your blood's level of "bad" cholesterol (low-density lipoprotein, or LDL), and lowers your level of "good" cholesterol (high-density lipoprotein, or HDL).

- Monounsaturated and polyunsaturated fats are found in plant foods such as vegetables, nuts, and grains, as well as oils made from these nuts and grains (canola, corn, and soybean). Omega-3 and omega-6 fatty acids are polyunsaturated. Besides vegetables, nuts, and grains, omega-3 and omega-6 fatty acids are found in coldwater fish such as tuna, salmon, and mackerel. Some studies have shown that eating foods that have mono or polyunsaturated fats can help reduce your levels of "bad" (LDL) cholesterol. Mono and polyunsaturated fats may also keep your triglyceride levels low. Triglycerides are a form of fat in your bloodstream. People with high triglyceride levels often have high total cholesterol, high LDL cholesterol, and low HDL ("good") cholesterol. Studies have linked high triglyceride levels to increased risk of stroke and heart disease.

Fats give you more concentrated calories than carbohydrates or proteins. In other words, a teaspoon of fat will have more calories than a teaspoon of carbs or a teaspoon of protein.

- Vitamins keep your bones strong, your vision clear and sharp, and your skin, nails, and hair healthy and glowing. Vitamins also help your body use energy from the food you eat.

- Minerals are chemical elements that help regulate your body's processes. Potassium, for example, helps your nerves and muscles function. Calcium helps your teeth and bones stay strong. Iron carries oxygen to your cells.

- If you eat a balanced diet with enough calories and protein, you are probably getting enough vitamins and minerals. However, if you are receiving treatment for breast cancer, this may be a challenge. In addition, certain treatments may sap your body's supplies of some vitamins or minerals.

- It is also important to remember that there is a big difference between getting your nutrients through food and taking supplements (vitamins, minerals, and herbals/botanicals). Vitamins and minerals work together in your body in very complex ways, affecting each other's absorption, processing, and influencing how your body functions. When you get your vitamins and minerals through eating foods, it is often easier for your body to maintain a balance of these nutrients. When you take a supplement, such as a vitamin C or E tablet, you are getting a highly concentrated dose that you would probably never get from food. While some supplements may be beneficial, others may reduce the effectiveness of certain breast cancer treatments.

- Water is necessary for life, which makes it vital for good health. Water makes up about half to two-thirds of your total body weight. It regulates your temperature, moves nutrients through your body, and gets rid of waste. During breast cancer treatment, you may experience diarrhea or vomiting. Losing all of these fluids plus the chemicals and minerals they contain can lead to dehydration.

- In general, it is a good idea to drink six to eight glasses of water a day. If you have lost fluids because of diarrhea or vomiting, you need to replace both the fluids and the essential ingredients in them. Chicken or vegetable broth, tomato juice, fruit juices, and Gatorade are examples of fluids that can help you replace the vitamins and minerals your body has lost.

14. Balancing Your Diet

To have a healthy, balanced diet, you need to eat a wide variety of foods from all the food groups.

Your best bet is to choose the most nutritionally rich foods you can from each food group each day—those packed with vitamins, minerals, fiber, and other nutrients, but also lower in calories. Pick foods like fruits, vegetables, whole grains, and fat-free or low-fat milk and milk products. You may want to choose organic sources of foods. (Organic means that no man-made pesticides, hormones, or antibiotics were applied to the crop while it was being grown or were applied to feed that was given to animals that provided the food, or were given to the animals.)

Figure Out How Many Calories You Need

What is the right number of calories for you to eat each day? This number depends on your age, health status, activity level, and whether you are trying to gain, maintain, or lose weight. You could use up all your calories on a few high-calorie items, but chances are you wouldn't get the full range of vitamins and nutrients your body needs to be healthy.

Knowing exactly how many calories your body needs per day can be an important first step in creating a healthy, balanced diet. The USDA Children's Nutrition Research Center at the Baylor College of Medicine has an online tool that will calculate the daily calories you need based on your sex, age, height, activity level, and weight. If you would like to weigh less than you do now, put in your desired weight and you'll see how many calories you need to get down to that weight.

You may want to talk to a registered dietitian about how to create a healthy diet plan that is right for you. You can get a list of dietitians in your ZIP code at the American Dietetic Association web site.

Analyze Your Diet

Counting calories and measuring nutrient levels are only a beginning. You may want to do more to design a diet that meets your individual goals. If you are unable to work directly with a registered dietitian, you have some other options. Computer programs and online tools can help you further analyze what you eat. They go beyond whether or not you are getting enough of a specific nutrient. Some of them might even make recommendations about how much of specific foods you should eat per day and track your eating and nutrient patterns over time.

Knowing What a Normal Portion Size Looks Like

After you decide how many calories, you need to eat per day, decide which foods you are going to eat, do not let super-sized portions ruin your good plans. Try to visualize the items below when you are planning a meal, ordering food out, or grabbing a snack.

For example, the USDA recommends you eat three to four ounces of meat, poultry, or fish as part of a healthy meal. That is about the size of a deck of cards. One study found that the typical portion size is at least twice as large, and some may be eight times as large! Reducing your portion size is a good step toward a healthy diet, even if you do not get down to the suggested portion sizes listed here. **Enjoy your food!**

Section 3

The Myths You Hear About Breast Cancer

15. The Myths about Breast Cancer

What you do not know CAN hurt you. Misinformation can keep you from recognizing and minimizing your own risk of breast cancer or getting the very best possible care. Arm yourself with the facts.

Here are ten common myths about breast cancer, followed by myths about specific types of breast cancer treatment.

1. Breast cancer only affects older women.

   Is this statement true? No.

   While it is true that the risk of breast cancer increases, as we grow older, breast cancer can occur at any age. From birth to age 39, one woman in 231 will get breast cancer (<0.5% risk); from age 40–59, the chance is one in 25-(4% risk); from age 60–79, the chance is one in 15 (nearly 7%). **Assuming you live to age 90**, the chance of getting breast cancer over the course of an entire lifetime is one in seven, with an overall lifetime risk of 14.3%.

2. If you have a risk factor for breast cancer, you are likely to get the disease.

   Is this statement true? No.

   Getting breast cancer is not a certainty, even if you have one of the stronger risk factors, like a breast cancer gene abnormality. Of women with a BRCA1 or BRCA2 inherited genetic abnormality, 40–80% will develop breast cancer over their lifetime; 20–60% will not. All other risk factors are associated with a much lower probability of being diagnosed with breast cancer.

3. If breast cancer does not run in your family, you will not get it.

Is this statement true? No.

Every woman has some risk of breast cancer. About 80% of women who get breast cancer have no known family history of the disease. Increasing age – just the wear and tear of living – is the biggest single risk factor for breast cancer. For those women who do have a family history of breast cancer, your risk may be elevated a little, a lot, or not at all. If you are concerned, discuss your family history with your physician or a genetic counselor. You may be worrying needlessly.

4. Only your mother's family history of breast cancer can affect your risk.

Is this statement true? No.

A history of breast cancer in your mother's OR your father's family will influence your risk equally. That is because half of your genes come from your mother, half from your father. However, a man with a breast cancer gene abnormality is less likely to develop breast cancer than a woman that has a similar gene. Therefore, if you want to learn more about your father's family history, you have to look mainly at the women on your father's side, not just the men.

5. Using antiperspirants causes breast cancer.

Is this statement true? No.

There is no evidence that the active ingredient in antiperspirants or reducing perspiration from the underarm area, influences breast cancer risk. The supposed link between breast cancer and antiperspirants is based on misinformation about anatomy and a misunderstanding of breast cancer.

6. Birth control pills cause breast cancer.

Is this statement true? No.

Modern day birth control pills contain a low dose of the hormones estrogen and progesterone. Many research studies show no association between birth control pills and an increased risk of breast cancer. However, one study that combined the results of many different studies did show an association between birth control pills and a very small increase in risk. The study also showed that this slight increase in risk decreased over time. Therefore, after 10 years, birth control pills were not associated with an increase in risk. Birth control pills also have benefits:

- decreasing ovarian and endometrial cancer risk,

- relieving menstrual disorders, pelvic inflammatory disease, and ovarian, and cysts, and

- Improving bone mineral density.

As with any medicine, you have to weigh the risks and benefits and decide what is best for YOU.

7. Eating high-fat foods causes breast cancer.

Is this statement true? No.

Several large studies have not been able to demonstrate a clear connection between eating high-fat foods and a higher risk of breast cancer. Ongoing studies are attempting to clarify this issue further. We can say that avoidance of high-fat foods is a healthy choice for other reasons: to lower the "bad" cholesterol (low-density lipoproteins), increase the "good" cholesterol (high-density lipoproteins); to make more room your diet for healthier foods, and to help you control your weight. Excess body weight, IS a risk factor for breast cancer, because the extra fat increases the production of estrogen outside the ovaries and adds to the overall level of estrogen in the body. If you are already overweight, or have a tendency to gain weight easily, avoiding high-fat foods is a good idea.

8. A monthly breast self-exam is the best way to diagnose breast cancer.

Is this statement true? No.

High quality, film-screen mammography is the most reliable way to find breast cancer as early as possible, when it is curable. By the time a breast cancer can be felt, it is usually bigger than the average size of a cancer first found on mammography. Breast examination by you or your healthcare provider is still very important. About 25% of breast cancers are found only on breast examination (not on the mammogram), about 35% are found on mammography alone, and 40% are found by both physical exam and mammography. Keep both bases covered.

9. I am at high risk for breast cancer and there is nothing I can do about it.

Is this statement true? No.

There are several effective ways to reduce—but not eliminate—the risk of breast cancer in women at high risk. Options include lifestyle changes (minimize alcohol consumption, stop smoking, exercise regularly), medication (tamoxifen, also called Nolvadex); and in cases of very high risk, surgery may be offered (prophylactic mastectomies, and for some women, prophylactic ovary removal). Be sure that you have consulted with a physician or genetic counselor before you make assumptions about your level of risk.

10. A breast cancer diagnosis is an automatic death sentence.

Is this statement true? No.

Fully 80% of women diagnosed with breast cancer have no signs of metastases (no cancer has spread beyond the breast and nearby lymph nodes). Furthermore, 80% of these women live at least five years, longer, and many live much longer. Even women with signs of cancer metastases can live a long time. In addition, promising treatment breakthroughs are becoming available each day.

16. The Myths about Breast Cancer Surgery

Many myths about breast cancer surgery have been passed from one generation of women to another. It is hard enough to deal with the reality of this disease, without worrying about things that are not true. In addition, it is important not to let those common misconceptions stand in the way of getting the best treatment available. Here are some of the most common myths about breast cancer surgery:

1. Surgery opens up the cancer to the air and makes it spread.

   Is this statement true? No.

   You are feeling just fine, and then something suspicious is discovered in your breast. Surgery is performed and the diagnosis comes back: cancer. When later tests show cancer elsewhere, you may immediately think that it was the surgery that released the cancer cells to the air, letting them jump all over the body ("After all, I couldn't feel them before"). However, metastatic breast cancer (cancer that has spread outside the breast to other areas of the body) can be silent for a long time before. The surgery did not cause the cancer to go elsewhere; it was there well before the surgery.

2. Mastectomy is safer than lumpectomy with radiation therapy.

   Is this statement true? Not necessarily true.

For women who have one site of breast cancer, with a tumor less than four centimeters that is removed with clear margins, lumpectomy with radiation is likely to be equally as effective as mastectomy.

3. If you have a strong history of breast cancer in your family, lumpectomy plus radiation is not for you.

Is this statement true? No.

Having breast cancer in your family does not mean that your cancer is automatically more threatening than anyone else's. It does not mean that breast-conserving therapy is not an option for you. You and your doctor will weigh several factors in deciding which type of surgery is right for you, based on:

1. your disease stage,

2. the cancer's "personality," and

3. How aggressive you want to be to prevent a recurrence or a new cancer from ever starting in that breast.

4. If your lymph nodes are removed, your arm will be swollen for the rest of your life.

Is this statement true? No.

Lymph node surgery can lead to uncomfortable side effects, including lingering discomfort, numbness, and swelling called lymphedema. Usually, this happens in only 5–10% of cases. The risk of lymphedema can approach the 25% level if you have a full axillary dissection, (levels I, II, and III of nodes removed) AND radiation was added to the lymph node areas after surgery, AND chemotherapy was given. Proper use and care of the affected arm, as well as physical therapy, can help manage lymphedema and reduce its severity.

17. The Myths about Radiation Therapy

It is natural for anyone beginning a new medical treatment to be a little fearful—or scared to death, depending on who you are. For women beginning radiation therapy, this fear seems to be heightened by some common misunderstandings about the treatment.

1. Radiation therapy is painful.

Is this statement true? Not really.

Most patients have no sensation of radiation when the machine is delivering the daily treatment. A few patients report a slight warming or tingling sensation in the area while the radiation machine is on. Over time, the skin in the area being treated will gradually become dry, sore, itchy, or burning. These feelings can be uncomfortable, but usually not enough for a woman to stop or interrupt her treatment.

2. Radiation therapy will cause me to be radioactive.

Is this statement true? Only in certain cases.

If you are treated with external radiation, you will not be radioactive at any time. The radiation you receive delivers its dose to your tissues within an instant—there is no lingering radiation once the treatment machine is turned off. As you try to keep to the normal rhythms of your life, it is important to remind friends, family, and co-workers that you will not expose them to radiation. If you receive internal radiation as a "boost" at the end of treatment, you will be radioactive while the radioactive material is in you. While you receive this internal treatment, you will be secluded in the hospital in a private room.

3. Radiation therapy will cause me to lose my hair.

Is this statement true? No. Not on your head, anyway.

If you are undergoing just radiation treatment, you will not lose the hair on your head (the hair on your nipple or in your lower armpit next to the breast might come out during radiation, but will grow back). The misperception that radiation makes you lose your hair comes from the confusion of radiation and chemotherapy. Since many patients begin radiation treatment right after their chemotherapy, it is understandable that the side effects of the two therapies are confused. Because chemotherapy is a "systemic" treatment, meaning it affects the whole body, you will likely lose your hair during this treatment. Radiation therapy is a "local" treatment, which means it is directly focused on the tissue of the breast area, and possibly nearby lymph nodes. Unless radiation is targeted at your head, you will not lose your hair from radiation.

4. Radiation therapy will cause nausea and vomiting.

Is this statement true? No.

Radiation treatment to the breast and lymph nodes will not cause nausea or vomiting. Most likely, this myth also arises from the common confusion of chemotherapy and radiation. Certain chemotherapy drugs may cause nausea and vomiting. In addition, medicines such as tamoxifen and certain pain medications can cause mild nausea. You also might find that your stomach becomes upset just from all the stress and anxiety of dealing with your illness.

5. Radiation therapy will increase my chance of getting more breast cancer.

Is this statement true? No.

The purpose of having breast radiation therapy is to reduce the risk of recurrence in that breast. Radiation to one breast does not increase your chance of getting cancer in the other breast. It is true that there is a relationship between radiation and cancer: Adolescent girls receiving chest radiation for Hodgkin's disease have a higher risk of getting breast cancer because the newly developing breast is especially vulnerable to radiation damage. In addition, a small percentage of women who were exposed to the atomic bomb blast at Hiroshima during World War II suffered from higher levels of breast cancer later in life. We now understand that this occurred because women were exposed to low levels of radiation over their entire body. The therapeutic radiation you will receive, however, is targeted precisely to the breast area, with almost no "scatter" to other areas of your body.

18. The Myths about Chemotherapy

1. The more chemotherapy you receive, the better you will do.

   Is this statement true? More is not necessarily better.

   When it comes to chemotherapy, the right combination of drugs is most important, not going beyond the standard dosage. Getting at least the standard dosage is very important, but going above that offers no real advantage.

2. If you do not get sick from chemotherapy, the treatment is not working.

   Is this statement true? No.

   The "no pain, no gain" rumors about chemotherapy are just that—rumors. There is no correlation between the amount that someone suffers from chemotherapy and the benefit it has against the cancer. Everyone responds differently. Some women have very few side effects; some have them daily.

3. Younger women have greater nausea on chemotherapy.

   Is this statement true? Yes.

   It is true. The younger you are, the more likely you are to be nauseated. Younger women have a larger nausea-trigger zone in the brain that decreases as you get old.

4. You have to get nauseated first, so the doctors will know how you respond to the chemotherapy.

Is this statement true? No.

No one has to get sick. Your first dose of anti-nausea medication will be given along with your chemotherapy, and you will have oral medication to take home with you to take for the first 48 hours.

5. You will be sicker with each chemotherapy treatment. In addition, you will be more exhausted as time goes on.

Is this statement true? Yes and No.

Your doctor or nurse should be able to adjust your supportive medications to help alleviate your symptoms if you are feeling sick after chemotherapy. Being sick after your first round does not necessarily mean you will be sick or sicker the next time. Fatigue is cumulative, though. You will not start to feel completely energetic again until the entire course of treatment is over.

Section 4
Self-Help Techniques

19. Your Inner Self

Every individual has his or her own beliefs. I believe that each person's life is predestined and what I mean by that is that God plans our lives before we are born. I feel that everything happens for a reason. You need to love everything about yourself and realize that God does everything for a reason. We may not understand now, but eventually our questions will be answered as time goes on.

This does not necessarily mean that the answers to our questions will be laid out on the table for you, but eventually you will put together the pieces to the puzzle. Yet as time passes, we can usually see things more clearly and comprehend why everything turned out the way it did. I feel that God walks with us during these troublesome times, and he gives us tools we need to get through these times. As these problems are occurring, we are learning also, so we can help others struggling. It is our decision to choose, if we are going to use the tools God has given us. Rejecting the options God has given us would be foolish because it will help better our lives and strengthen our inner souls.

Each individual has three parts, the mind, body and spirit. We can do anything we put our minds too. The mind is a powerful and vital part of our body. Many underestimate its capability.

Accepting that you have breast cancer, realizing what is ahead and the obstacles that need to be dealt with are the most important and most critical step in learning to cope with breast cancer. To live with a happy state of mind, you need to have high self-esteem. You need to feel that you are no different from anyone else and that you can be the person you set in your mind to be. You need to reconstruct your life. You need to put yourself in a lifestyle that will make you happy and bring you as little stress as possible.

Stress is the worst thing for someone with breast cancer. You have enough of stress dealing with breast cancer, do not let the other things in life stress you. There are more important things in your life you need to conquer.

Therefore, you most try to avoid stressful situations and try to live your life with as little stress possible. During the day if you feel stressed, you should try massage therapy. This is when you relax the muscles, ease muscle spasms and pain, increase blood flow in the skin and muscles, relieve mental and emotional stress, and induce relaxation.

You could also try listening to music to relieve stress or talk to someone about what is bothering you. Having a pet aids in reducing stress. If you tend to stress easily, you may want to give some thought to having an animal friend to help reduce your stress.

Learning to love everything about yourself is one major step in learning to accept that you have breast cancer. If you are unhappy with yourself, then you need to change what makes you unhappy by going through the process of change.

The process of change involves several things. First, let us ask ourselves, what does loving ourselves for who we are really mean? What does it involve? Is this something that is easy to accomplish or does it take time and effort? Learning to love ourselves is not easy and it does not happen overnight. Loving yourself takes time and this is something you must work at each day. You need to be able to get up each morning, and look in the mirror and like the person that you see. If you are unhappy with that person than you have to do something about it.

I have worked hard trying to change the things that I did not like about myself. It has taken me years of hard work to get to this point. I realize that I am no different from anyone else. I do not feel embarrassed about having epilepsy and have become the person I set forth to be. Nevertheless, the key to all this is living life with a healthy and productive perspective, not a rebellious one. You must set reasonable goals and objectives in your life.

The first thing, I did to help me on my road to success was to say to myself aloud, "I am Stacey Chillemi and yes, I have a seizure disorder." You need to hear yourself say that there is nothing is wrong with having breast cancer, absorb it into your unconscious and conscious mind.

Once you learn to strengthen your inner self and develop strong self-esteem, you will begin to feel you can accomplish whatever you set your mind on. You must understand and truly believe that no one can change you; only you can change yourself.

I learned to love myself by accepting all my faults and putting the past behind me, but if, you focus on your faults than you will only experience an unhappy life. You need to think positively and focus on your accomplishments.

My life began to change for the better once I started to focus on my achievements and stopped dwelling on negative things. We all deserve to live life to its fullest.

To be able to live with breast cancer, you need to develop a great emotional strength so you can accept the negative things about yourself, yet want to change them. To heal yourself you must focus on all your positive qualities. You must change the factors that lessen your self-worth. Doing so will help you live a happy and healthy life and make you feel that you can accomplish anything the world dishes out to you.

To begin the healing process we need to develop strength, wisdom, confidence and knowledge. If you can develop these qualities, you will achieve all your goals and dreams. First, you must focus on the goals and dreams you want to fulfill. I am going to teach you the true meaning of strength, wisdom, confidence, and knowledge. I will show you how to obtain them and how to use them. This process of change theory will help you live a happy life and you will not be ashamed that you have breast cancer.

Understand that all these characteristics come from inside us. Have you ever heard the expression, "mind over matter?" It means learning to take control of yourself and the world around you by using the knowledge you have gained. To use your mind productively, you have to understand yourself. The people who do not let others take control of them are the individuals who know what is best for them. By developing and acting on these qualities, you can look at breast cancer in a positive way and not view it as the ruination of your life. You are probably thinking, "What!" "Is this chick crazy?" No, I am not!" You need to take charge of yourself and learn how to nurture yourself. You cannot hide the fact that you have breast cancer, and should not. You must become proud of who you are and realize that you are not the only one with breast cancer. Millions go through it each year and overcome it, and they become one of the millions of breast cancer survivors.

Now let us look at each individual characteristic separately.
Strength—the development of strength in the inner body begins in the mind. The inner body is our mind, soul and spirit. How we think and program our minds to work, helps us build mental, physical and spiritual strength. Our strength comes from how we feel about ourselves. The higher our self-esteem, the stronger we feel and in turn, we can do more for ourselves.

I cannot even begin to stress the importance of having high self-esteem; it is the key to having mental, physical and spiritual strength. The first stage of developing strength is learning to love yourself and your life. You need to learn to be grateful for what God has given you. You need to let go of all those angry emotions inside. Holding anger inside yourself will not help you, it will only hurt you. The past is just that— over. There is no way of changing the fact that you have or had breast cancer. Yet, if you have the strength and motivation, you can make the present anything you want.

Breast cancer will not interfere with your life unless, you let it. So many people who have written to me or people I have spoken to, felt angry because they have a disorder or a disease. To free yourself that anger, you have to say to yourself, "Yes, I have breast cancer. I accept the fact that I have breast cancer and that I am unable to change the past. Nevertheless, I can change my future because I love myself and refuse to hurt myself by drowning in my own self pity." You cannot rely on others. You need to learn to rely on yourself.

You have to believe in yourself, develop a sense of pride in yourself. It does not matter what others think about you, what matters is how you think about yourself. God put us on this earth to love ourselves and other people. He did not put us here to hurt ourselves and take our anger out on others, who are usually on the people we care about the most.

Knowledge—is the second part of the process of change; it is another important factor in helping deal with epilepsy. Knowledge comes from experience, from being open minded to suggestions others may give. We may not always agree with other people's suggestions, yet it is always wise to listen to what others have to say. Some individuals may try to be controlling and may get frustrated if we do not act on what they have to say. You should set these people straight and tell them; I will listen to what you have to say; however, that does not necessarily mean I am going to agree with you. I have my own mind, too and I need to do what is best for me.

We learn from each other and we acquire knowledge from the world around us that we should pass along to others by helping them. We need to take our experience and use it in our present life now, including the mistakes we have made in life. The mistakes we have made are where we get most of our knowledge that helps us become stronger individuals. What weakens us when we repeatedly make the same mistakes?

Do not pity yourself for the mistakes you made in life or imperfections. Studies have shown that people who have negative attitudes are more likely to live chaotic lives. They are more likely to become mentally or physically ill with extremely debilitating or life threatening illnesses. Many people have a hard time focusing on the positive because they allow their negative sides to consume them... I firmly believe that focusing on the negatives will causes seizures.

Say to yourself, OK, what I have learned from these mistakes or from my shortcomings. Taking what you have learned and using it to help others is the best therapy. When you help, you feel a sense of accomplishment and self-worth. You are overlooking any negative characteristics because you are too busy focusing on helping others'.

Confidence—our confidence comes from our self-esteem. To have high self-esteem we need to feel good about ourselves, to get to this point in life you need to begin by starting to do things in life to make yourself happy by focusing on the future, creating direction in your life. Begin by planning short and long-term goals for yourself and confidence level will rise.

It worked for me. When I started accomplishing some of my short-term goals, I had more self-respect. I developed a greater sense of pride and my inner strength and self-worth increased.

Wisdom—comes from your sixth sense. We all have five senses, our sight, hearing, smell, taste, touch, yet I believe wisdom to be our sixth sense. The meaning of wisdom is to be able to understand your inner signals and the answers that your body sends out to you, becoming aware of what your body is trying to tell you. Your sixth sense always leads you to the right answers. It is up to us to learn to understand our inner self (spirit) and to follow the signals it sends out to us.

Listening to what our inner self has to say is essential. For example, have you ever felt like you had a feeling something was the right thing to do? You need to learn to understand your mind, so you can understand your inner soul and all the wonderful things our soul is capable of doing. When we listen and act on signals our inner self-gives us, we become stronger. Slowly, we begin to understand our body as a whole. Spiritually you can give your body what it needs.

We feed our body food to survive on a daily basis. Spiritually we need to feed our body with love, understanding and different forms of relaxation, such as meditation. I strongly suggest that everyone starts with relaxation exercise for al least five minutes daily.

Either in the morning when you start your day, the afternoon if you are able to, or at night before bed. This will help to release the tension that has built up throughout the day. Each week you should add five minutes until you get to an hour each day.

When you do these things, you increase your level of strength, wisdom, knowledge and confidence. By having a high level of strength you feel as though, you can conquer the world. This helps you decrease your stress level.

Once you accept your breast cancer in your life, you can cope with the world around you and accept the fact that you can do everything you expected to do in life. However, to accept that you have breast cancer you first have to love who you are and be proud of the person you have become. There are many things in life you are capable of doing, but you must develop the motivation and the will to get out there and **JUST DO THEM**!

20. Creating the New You

Changing yourself mentally, physically and spiritually does not happen overnight. The process of change takes much time and energy, so do not get discouraged. While focusing on this program you will begin to see the changes in yourself as they start to occur. I felt exceptionally proud of myself when I saw myself begin to change for the better. My self-esteem improved and I no longer cared what others thought about me. For the first time I was concerned about what I thought, not what others thought.

Believe me, once you begin working on this program you will begin seeing results and realize that this program is worth doing.

Remember, you cannot say you want to change; you have really to want it to do it. The motivation to want to change has to come from within your heart. Saying you want to change is easy, but you have really to want it to do it for it to happen. Otherwise, the change will never occur.

Below, are the seven steps to the, "beginning of the transformation process." The transformation process begins when you realize it is time to change and you finally develop the stamina to do what it takes to improve yourself. I created seven steps so that starting the program the right way will be easier for you. Your mind, body and soul all have to be on the same track, functioning as one or else the program will not work for you. The most important part of the program is the beginning. You have to have the correct perception of what you will be doing now and where you will be headed for the future.

I used these seven steps myself to help me change my outlook my life. I was able love myself and not be ashamed that I had disorder. In addition, you should not be ashamed that you have breast cancer. I felt capable of living the life the way I wanted too. I felt like a different, person. I strongly believe that if you follow the techniques in this book that it will help to live your life in a positive manner and if you have breast cancer these techniques will give you the strength to cope with your breast cancer.

Below are the seven steps to help you get on with your life.

STEP ONE:

PATIENCE—the first step to help you to look at live in a positive manner is to develop patience. You will need patience to work this program successfully. Changing your outlook on life is going to take time, devotion and hard work. Succeeding with this program comes by being patient in wanting to see results.

The following exercise will help you even if you are already a patient person because it will relax you and increase your motivational skills simultaneously.

1. Take a warm bubble bath for fifteen minutes. Also, place an oatmeal bath in the water.

2. Lie in the bathtub and close your eyes, take four deep breaths slowly.

3. While you are taking these deep breaths clear all thoughts from your mind. Focus on the feeling of the warm water touching your body and the breathing techniques that you are doing at that moment.

4. Think about something positive and pleasant. Envision something that makes you happy. Focus on something that makes you feel good about yourself.

5. Let go of any negative thoughts that you have stored in your mind. Just think about one thing that makes you feel good about yourself.

6. Take four more deep breaths, relax for a minute and get out of the bathtub.

7. Get dressed, go to a quiet place and sit on the floor. Close your eyes and slowly bend forward, relaxing

any tight muscles that are causing you tension. Bend to the left, stretching your arms as far as they will go, then stretch to the right, repeating the movement.

8. Take five more deep breaths and say aloud "I have the patience to change myself and become the person I want to become in life." Say, "I have breast cancer and there is nothing wrong with that."

9. Repeat step seven and eight

10. Take five more deep breaths and listen to yourself when you are doing this exercise. Concentrate on yourself while doing this exercise. Do not let any distractions impose on your quiet time. Do not think about anything except this exercise and the techniques it involves. Changing your outlook on breast cancer means to not let your breast cancer take control of you. As I was growing up, I always made believe that I did not have epilepsy. By doing this, I was only hurting myself. Accepting my disorder into my life has helped me tremendously. I have released much of the anger that I held inside myself, and have focused on other parts of my life. As a result, I have become a stronger person, extremely proud of the person I have become. You need to do the same. It may take time to get to this point. That is why you need to have patience and believe you can do anything you put your mind to. Thinking positive thoughts about yourself will help you get a long way in life.

STEP TWO:

This step teaches you how to recognize all the wonderful things about yourself. Judging other people is very easy. Looking at ourselves honestly, however, is difficult. Sometimes we do not focus on ourselves because we have become so preoccupied focusing on everyone else that we forget number one. This step helps recognize all the good things about you. You will begin to have a more positive outlook on life. First, you need to ask, "What do I have to change about myself? What parts of my life need to change? What are my strengths? What are my weaknesses?

Before you answer these questions, get yourself a notebook to document your answers to these questions and keep track of your progress. The journal helps you see your characteristics and change the ones you dislike. Look at the positive things about yourself and commend yourself for the accomplishments that you achieved and work on changing the negative characteristics that we all carry within us. Begin the journal by listing all the positive things about yourself on the first page. Make a list that looks like the following.

Example:

THE POSITIVE THINGS ABOUT ME

Strengths

1.
2.
3.
4.
5.
6.
7.
8.
9.
10.

Your positive points are the strengths that will take you through life. Start your journal with these positive characteristics about yourself. Seeing your strengths itemized in your daily journal will give you encouragement. Each day as you open this journal, you will be looking at all the good things about yourself that will give you motivation to make this program help you achieve your highest potential. On the next page, create a list and write down your weaknesses. Make a list that looks as the following. Remember, be honest with yourself and make sure you focus not only on your strengths, but also on your weaknesses. Reviewing our weaknesses can help us see more clearly, what has to change in our lives.

THE THINGS ABOUT MYSELF THAT I NEED TO WORK ON

Weaknesses

1.
2.
3.
4.
5.
6.
7.
8.
9.
10.

On the next page, list ten goals you want to do this week to change your outlook on epilepsy and how you feel about yourself. This will help you gain some insight into what you need to start doing for yourself. Start planning what you want the new you to be like. Each time you accomplish a goal, put a star next to it. Write down the date of when you achieved the goal.

Create a list that looks like the following:

Example:

MAKING THE NEW ME

Goals for the Week /Date

1. I wrote a letter to five people with breast cancer. * 9/15
2.
3.
4.
5.
6.
7.
8.
9.
10.

Then I want you to list ten long-term goals of what you want to have accomplished and where you want to be in a month's time. Focus on how you are going to accept your breast cancer, be proud of yourself. Focus on how you are going to change the characteristics about yourself that you do not like. *Make the list look like the list I have created below for you:*

CREATING THE NEW ME

Goals for the Month

1.
2.
3.
4.
5.
6.
7.
8.
9.
10.

Create a page in the beginning of the book called the PRIORITY CALENDAR. Ask your self these questions.

PRIORITY CALENDAR

What do you regret not having made more time for?

1.
2.
3.
4.
5.
6.
7.
8.
9.
10.

If you had more time, what would you do with it?

1.
2.
3.
4.

5.
6.
7.
8.
9.
10.

What are the top ten priorities in your life right now?

1.
2.
3.
4.
5.
6.
7.
8.
9.
10.

What are your family-related goals?

1.
2.
3.
4.
5.
6.
7.
8.
9.
10.

What are your business goals?

1.
2.
3.
4.
5.
6.
7.
8.
9.
10.

In the back of the journal, take a quarter of the notebook and title it your Daily Diary. Dedicate the diary to someone you care about and feel close to, someone who would be proud to see you accepting that you have breast cancer and to see that you are moving forward.

Dedicate this journal to someone; you care about because it gives you motivation to want to become a better person. Write about the goals you accomplished and explain how it made you feel to reach them. Write about how these achievements are making you into a better person and how they are helping you with your recovery. Describe what you had to do to achieve the goals.

Example:

Date

STEP THREE:

This step is about the importance of self-determination. This step will show you how to develop self-determination. Self-determination comes from with-in. Self-determination requires that you make an agreement with yourself and keep it. You must have faith in yourself that you are going to do anything that you put your mind too. Your motivation to accomplish this program will become easier as each day goes by. Saying you are going to improve is easy, but you cannot just say you are going to improve; you have to get out and accomplish the goals that you have set for yourself. You cannot accomplish too many goals in one day. Changing takes time and as step one says, "You need to have patience." Try to accomplish one goal a week at first. Maybe two goals, if you have the time.

Accomplish a different goal each week until you get to ten goals. These goals do not have to be difficult. You can set several little goals or maybe only one large one. Working on yourself can be tough if you have a busy schedule; nevertheless, do not let that stop you. You have to make time for yourself. Remember, you come first in life. You need to believe that you are the best. You cannot take care of the people who mean the most to you or do the things in life that you want to do, if you are mental, physical and spiritual well-being is not intact and strong.

STEP FOUR:

Reward yourself every time you achieve a goal. Your achievements are important and you should not treat them lightly. For example, take in a movie or reward yourself with some quiet time to relax and focus just on yourself. To me there is nothing better than having some "ME TIME" this means being alone. Taking some time-out for yourself. Do something that makes you happy. Remember, you cannot make others happy until you are happy with yourself.

STEP FIVE:

In your journal, make a list called, "Record of Successes" and itemize all the achievements that you have accomplished. Create a list of everything good you believe you have done for yourself. This will make you feel good about yourself. For example, include the following:

RECORD OF SUCCESSES THROUGHOUT MY LIFE

My Achievements

1.
2.
3.
4.
5.
6.
7.
8.
9.
10.

RECORD OF SUCCESSES DURING THIS PROGRAM

My Achievements

1.
2.
3.
4.
5.
6.
7.
8.
10.

STEP SIX:

Develop a special time in the day for quiet time. Studies have shown that individuals who have a daily quiet time are less likely to become ill, and heal faster from illness than those who do not. Take a few minutes during the day to write in your journal. Try to make it the same time each day.

Perhaps, when no one is home or in the morning, just before you start the day. You could also wait until everyone goes to sleep so that no one will bother you. Give yourself at least fifteen minutes to a half hour. Relax, and while you are writing and relaxing ask yourself the question: "Where am I headed in life and where do I want to be a year from now?" Then write about it. Make sure you are focusing on the things you want to accomplish in life.

The only way you will succeed in this life is making sure that epilepsy does not control your life. You need to feel proud of the changes you are making with this program. Focus on what you have accomplished. Think about how you feel about having breast cancer as you write in this journal.

The goal is to let yourself open up and write intimately and honestly about how you feel. This method helps heal your wounds so you can get on with your life. You have to learn to understand why you have reacted the way you have about having breast cancer. Think of ways to strengthen yourself spiritually and emotionally. Make sure you do not limit yourself because you feel sorry for yourself because you have breast cancer. This is self-pity and it is extremely unhealthy mentally, physically and spiritually. You will never get anywhere in life if you pity yourself. Free yourself from any walls you have built around yourself. This program will help you do that. Become the person you were destined to become.

STEP SEVEN:

Now repeat the seven-step process each day. Once you complete the seven steps go back and review the things you have written in your journal. These steps are a new way of life. Keep doing these seven steps each day until you get to where you want to be and you have become completely satisfied with yourself. There is so much knowledge out there for us to learn. It is there for anyone who wants it. I always add more goals to my list. You should always work on bettering yourself. Everyone is special. Everyone has something unique about him or her. It is your job to find out what those unique qualities are in you and how to make them work for you.

21. Being Honest With Yourself

The only way to succeed in this program or in life is to be honest with yourself. Have you been trying to hide the fact that you have breast cancer? Are you in denial? If so, it is time to let go of your fears, your shame and accept who you are. If you have been carrying many angry feelings inside yourself because you are angry about having breast cancer, then you must rid yourself of those angry feelings.

Often when we carry angry feelings inside ourselves, we take them out on those around us. We also hide our weaknesses and the things we do not like about ourselves from others, hide them and from ourselves. As a result, all the negative characteristics and emotions that we do not fix now will eat away at us little by little, and the person who suffers the most is you. Be honest with yourself so you can heal your old wounds and begin a new way of life with a clean slate.

Lying to yourself and to the people around you will get you nowhere in this life. You will get farther in life by being honest with yourself and others. There is no such thing as telling little white lies. One lie leads to another lie, and the lie grows bigger. Being honest with yourself is not something you do just in this program; you must be honest throughout your life.

You have to be proud of yourself. If there is something about yourself you are not happy with, then you need to change it. To do this, you must be honest with yourself.

Breast cancer is a part of your life. It will not disappear, so you need to learn how to live a fulfilling life. Understand that you are not alone and that there are many individuals with the same condition. These individuals are eagerly looking for support. Breast Cancer should not stop you from accomplishing what you want in life, unless you let it.

Our main goal is to repair all the emotional and psychological damage that we have inflicted upon ourselves over the years that have been harmful to our mind, body and soul. Say that, "I am not going to hurt myself like this anymore. I am too good a person for this." You are who you make yourself to be. To feel better you must free yourself from the entire negative ness that you stored inside yourself and fill your soul with peace and serenity.

You cannot and should not blame anyone for your breast cancer. Rid yourself of any resentment you maybe carrying toward yourself. Make your condition a part of yourself. For many years, I have kept this saying in my mind. Maybe it will help you:

God grant me the serenity to accept the things I cannot change

The courage to change the things I can

And the wisdom to know the difference

22. Your Dreams Are Not Just Dreams – The True Meaning of Dreams

Dreams are the pathways to our inner souls that come from our subconscious mind. While we are sleeping, our body tries to send us messages about the wants and needs our body. A person's dreams can give a sense of direction in life. Although we do not remember most of our dreams when we wake up, they still have an impact on the way we think and function.

Sigmund Freud believed that dreams are expressions of unfulfilled wishes and desires. Dreaming plays an important role in our lives. Speaking for myself, dreaming always helped me escape from reality to a faraway make believe world where no one could hurt me.

Studies have shown that people who are awakened repeatedly at the beginning of dream periods for several nights become irritable and have difficulty concentrating. If your body is natural sleep cycle has been interrupted and has been deprived of dream sleep, your body will compensate by providing proportionately more dream sleep at the next dream sleep opportunity. Research shows that a healthy sleep is needed for a person's body to restore itself. Some scientists believe that adequate dream sleep is equally important because it enables the brain to recharge. Medical research has not proven this testimony. Usually, when a person is awake, their brain waves will show a regular rhythm. When a person first falls asleep, the brain waves become slower and less regular. They call this sleep state non-rapid eye movement (NREM) sleep.

Sleep consists of stages. There are four stages and each stage is a progressively deeper stage. The deeper the sleep, the more your body restores itself. Stage one sleep is the transition from wakefulness to sleep. Restoration begins in stage two, but is more significant in stages three and four, sometimes called delta sleep.

After an hour and a half of NREM sleep, the brain waves begin to show a more active pattern again, though the individual is in a deep sleep. This sleep state, called rapid eye movement (REM) sleep, and is when dreaming occurs. A person typically experiences a brief arousal from sleep and returns to stage two sleep after dreaming. This sleep cycle has begun again. The length of time in each of these stages differs throughout the night, with most REM sleep occurring during the later sleep cycle.

Dreaming and fantasizing give you a feeling of serenity and inner peace. Fantasizing has a positive impact on you and your body. When you fantasize, you put yourself in a state of consciousness that lies between reality and the world of dreams. The imagination roams freely, although usually guided by mostly unconscious urges, concerns and memories. Fantasies help us find out what type of ambition we have and the people we want to become in life; it takes us into another world where we can do and become anything we want. It allows us to relax and joyfully think about the various scenarios that would make us happy.

While growing up, I always enjoyed sitting closing my eyes and fantasizing about something relaxing trying to analyze how my body was feeling the same time. It seemed when I understood my body and mind, I was able to make them function as one and then release all negative thoughts and feelings that was putting unnecessary stress on me. (Remember, the less stress you have the better for your condition.) Stress has a huge impact of your health.

During this time of dreaming and fantasizing, you can focus on anything you want, including making goals for yourself on how you are going to live your life having breast cancer and the fear that it could come back. I have always dreamed about positive things. I knew I was going to survive having epilepsy because I refused to think negatively or feel sorry for myself. I looked at myself as a fighter and an achiever. I was not going to let anything get in my way.

Dreams can stay in your mind, no one has to know about them, and you can record them, in your daily diary, where you write down your significant dreams and fantasies. These dreams and fantasies can be used as motivators to help you work on accepting epilepsy in your life and learning how to live with it. Your dreams and fantasies can help you plan your life five or even ten years from now and you can use your dreams to strengthen your inner self. When life seems too stressful to handle, close your eyes and let your mind take you somewhere you can relax and fantasize.

Dreams are the pathways to your inner soul and it is your soul that knows what your mind and body need. Reach out and get in contact with your soul because it is necessary that you take the time out to understand what your mind and body crave.

Keeping a journal has been a very successful tool for me. I write everything down on paper from my short-term goals to my long-term goals, to my dreams and fantasies. This helps increase my inner strength by keeping me in touch with who I am and what I need to do with my life. I write down everything about the exams I take, about switching my medicines and anything else that is important to me. By writing everything down and expressing how you feel emotionally you can understand yourself better and the needs of your mind, body, and soul.

The exercises you do in your journal will help you strengthen and understand yourself, and make you feel better about yourself as a person.

MY DREAMS

Date

1. WHAT THIS DREAM MEANT TO ME
2. HOW WILL I USE THIS DREAM TO MOTIVATE ME?

MY FANTASY

Date

1. WHAT THIS FANTASY MEANT TO ME
2. HOW WILL I USE THIS FANTASY TO MOTIVATE ME?

Keep a list of the dreams and fantasies you have that mean something special to you. Write down how they can motivate you in this program and how they relate to helping your breast cancer.

Do they relax you? Do they help increase your understandings of yourself better? Do they give you hope for the future? While you write in the dream portion of your journal, answer the questions above. This is another way to strengthen yourself and understand your personal make up. These exercises will help strengthen your mind, body and soul in many ways.

23. The Importance of Self-Esteem & Self-Confidence

High self-esteem and your strong self-confidence will get you far in life. If you believe in yourself then you can succeed in anything you put your mind to. You may not succeed the first time you try, but you have to keep trying until you do succeed. You are too good a person to let yourself get to that point. God has blessed you by giving you a life to live; now you need to make the best of it. People give up hope when they attempt new methods and programs and they do not improve quickly. I have learned from my own experience and from others whom I corresponded with that when you keep trying and you feel like you are not, ahead of where you have started, you begin to lose hope for the future. Quick success does not exist in our society.

This is when you need to use your strength and tell yourself to stop, that you are not going to pity yourself anymore. I battled with myself; sometimes I felt like I was winning the battle and at times I felt as though I would never make it over the hump, until one day I said, "no more." I was not going to feel like this anymore. From then on, my life had a drastic turnaround. I became determined to become a new person, filled with hope, who was going accomplish anything I set my mind to do.

Achievements only come to those who strive hard to get them. You get nowhere in life if you do not push yourself. You need to create a lifestyle that is right for you and nobody else. Do not settle for anyone else's lifestyle or for a lifestyle that is beneath your standards.

To make this happen, you must learn to accept who you, be proud of the person you are. Only then will you feel your self-esteem rise up to the skies'!

If you're still feeling that you don't have what it takes to complete this program then write whatever is still making you feel like you are not worthy of yourself in your journal. Even after completing the other exercises, if you still face obstacles that are holding you back, write them down in the journal immediately. Ask yourself what is making you feel like you cannot get to the point in life you want to reach. Organize your journal to look like this and write your feelings on the topics I just mentioned.

SELF-ESTEEM & SELF CONFIDENCE

1.
2.
3.
4.
5.
6.
7.
8.
9.
10.

Remember the past is over; you can only change the future. Having expressed what is bothering you, what you are holding you back, begin to think how you can change the way you feel. Go through your journal and look at all the positive things about yourself. Concentrate on your strengths. Write about why you do all the good things you do for yourself and for others in the back of your journal. These are the reasons you should love yourself and have high self-esteem and self-confidence in yourself. Give yourself credit for everything positive you have written about yourself. Remember, you are somebody special.

Ask yourself the question, what level of self-approval have I reached living with epilepsy on a day-to-day basis? I have listed seven levels. Each of these levels will help you see the daily progress that you are making with this program.

- **LEVEL 1**-accept yourself as someone with breast cancer and learn to love yourself for whom you are
- **LEVEL 2**-understand yourself mentally, physically and spiritually
- **LEVEL 3**-learn to control your mind, body and emotions

- **LEVEL 4**-strengthen your inner self and make it apparent to others
- **LEVEL 5**-begin changing what you do not like about yourself
- **LEVEL 6**-notice the change in your self-esteem and self-confidence
- **LEVEL 7**-have a tremendous amount of pride in yourself

When I went to the doctor for my illness, he would tell me what I could and could not do. I would become very frustrated. I would think to myself, "Leave me alone." You know medically what I go through, but you do are nit experiencing what I am going through, so how can you really understand what I am going through? When I would come home, my dad would make sure that I took care of myself. I was so sick of being looked after; I just wanted to be left alone. I know they were looking out for my best interest, but I had enough.

When I finally accepted myself as someone with my illness, I saw myself change one hundred percent. I became proud of myself. I saw myself no different from anyone else. I take my medicine. Some people take antidepressants. Other people take vitamins during the day. When I accepted that, I had an illness and suddenly began to love myself for who I was and focused on what I could be. This was the best thing I ever did for myself. I felt as free as the birds that fly in our beautiful skies.

I was no longer embarrassed of myself and I was finally facing my illness head on. A heavy accumulation of stress, depression and frustration left my body. Remember, there is nothing wrong with having breast cancer. You are a wonderful person will magnificent qualities to share with the world.

Accepting that is the most important and most critical step in learning to live with your disease. To live with a happy state of mind, you need to have high self-esteem. You need to feel that you are no different from anyone else. You need to reconstruct your life and create a lifestyle that will make you happy and bring you as little stress as possible.

Stress is the worst thing for someone with an illness. Stress can destroy you. Therefore, you most try to avoid stressful situations and try to live your life with as little stress possible. During the day if you feel you feel stressed, you should try massage therapy. This relaxes the muscles, eases muscle spasms and pain, increases blood flow in the skin and muscles and relieves mental and emotional stress, and induces relaxation. Also, try listening to music to relieve stress or talk to someone about what is bothering you. If you tend to stress easily, you may want to give some thought to having a pet to relax you. Everyone goes through life having to deal with something. You will survive. You shall overcome.

24. Using Mediation to Help You Cope with Breast Cancer

Mediation can be achieved in many ways. One way is to let your mind rest in open awareness. Let us begin…

When you mediate, you do not have to be focused to achieve the benefits of mediation. You can rest the mind naturally, through total awareness. Some people who practice mediation may ask, "What is she talking about? How am I suppose to rest my mind without focusing on a serene or relaxing image in my mind?"

You can rest your mind, by sitting in a bath, letting out a sigh, and just relaxing in an area in your home that a positive, relaxed, calm energy. This time is called your alone time. There is no standing on your feet, no work clothes on your body, just something that is comfortable. At this point, you need to say goodbye to all your worries. Do not think about work or any responsibilities you need to tackle. And most of all no TV or the computer!

This is how you rest yourself in objectless mediation. You need to just let go and relax. You do not have to stop of block whatever thoughts or emotions that enter your mind, but you do not have to focus on them or follow them. Let yourself rest, simply allowing whatever to occur. If thoughts and emotions come, let them, be aware of them just do not follow or focus on them. This is called, *"Objectless Shinay Mediation."*

Objectless Shinay Mediation does not mean letting you mind wonder without direction or putting your mind in fantasies. There is still some presence. This is called center of awareness. You are not focused on anything in particular, but you are still aware. You are aware of what is happening around you.

When you do this, you are resting the mind in its natural simplicity, different from focusing on thoughts and emotions.   This is kind of like accepting whatever comes your way, such as accepting whatever ocean wave comes to you. Recognizing that the ocean remains unchanged even though some waves are large and some are small. The ocean waters are always blue and always in motion.

In the same way, this mediation is always clear even when thoughts and emotions pop-up. All the simplicity, clearness, compassion, and calmness are enclosed within that state.

Other Techniques to Help You Relax When You Are Feeling Stressed

Relaxation techniques to help you learn how to relax and improve your relationship with time.

In today's world, time and stress play a big role in everyone's lives. It is amazing how simple life seemed in the 1950's compared to now.   Between work, family, and outside responsibilities when do we have time for ourselves? How many people can actually say that they are able to schedule a fair amount of me time into their schedule where they are able to pamper themselves and release all excess stress that has built up inside yourself. As time goes on you end up feeling like your ready to explode.

For people who want to help themselves relax, but are unfamiliar with all the different relation techniques I am going to show you techniques that you can practice in public or the privacy of your own home.

First, you need to need to learn how to incorporate daily relaxation steps in to your daily routine that are simple, quick, and easy to do.

You have been at work for hours - sitting at your office desk, staring into the computer, your eyes are stress out, your back is aching, your neck is tightening and you can feel the knots in your neck accumulating. Sound familiar?

When you feel like this you are probably thinking to yourself, "I wish I knew some relaxation techniques that I could do at my desk to help me relax, and also, relieve my stress and tensions from this job." You look at the clock your work is not completed yet your thinking when do I have get time for myself? Now's the time with the techniques listed below:

1. First, no matter what your job is everyone needs to take small breaks to give yourself a breather. Small breaks will re-energize you and help you become more focus. You cannot do a good job if you are not focused.

People often find themselves hunching over with their heads forward at their desk, chins sticking out, chest closed down. Using a few yoga poses, you can increase body awareness and prevent physical problems- such as degenerative disk disease and repetitive strain injuries- that can result from poor sitting habits. Practice these yoga positions at work or at home to help you recover from that terrible illness called "breast cancer - stress caused by your illness."

Tadasana (mountain Pose)

In many series of Yoga Exercises, Tadasana is a position used at the beginning, in the middle, and in the end, in which you pay attention to your position, your concentration and your breathing. During intensive Yoga sessions, Tadasana makes it easier for you to maintain your meditative focus, as well as to increase and regain it.

1. Stand up straight with both feet at hip-width.
2. Turn your heels a little outward and let your weight rest on your toes.
3. Your arms hang downwards along your body and the palm of your hands point towards your body.
4. Now make the back of your pelvis move away from your lower back. You can do this by drawing in your ribs a little in the direction of your belly.

5. Breathe in and out a few times with full concentration. Through your breathing, place your neck straight over the upper back. It would then feel as if you stretch your body upwards from the neck.
6. The shoulders feel broad and are relaxed.
7. Your breathing is free and relaxed.
8. Look straight ahead of you at a spot within your vision and try to stand motionless with as little effort as possible.
9. Whenever you do this exercise, do it with care and always try to increase your focus and your relaxation.

Garundasana (Eagle Pose)

The word is usually translated into English as "eagle," though according to one dictionary the name literally means "devourer," because Garuda was originally identified with the "all-consuming fire of the sun's rays."

Steps

1. Stand, bend your knees slightly, lift your left foot up and, balancing on your right foot, cross your left thigh over the right. Point your left toes toward the floor, press the foot back, and then hook the top of the foot behind the lower right calf. Balance on the right foot.

2. Stretch your arms straightforward, parallel to the floor, and spread your scapulas wide across the back of your torso. Cross the arms in front of your torso so that the right arm is above the left, and then bend your elbows. Snug the right elbow into the crook of the left, and raise the forearms perpendicular to the floor. The backs of your hands should be facing each other.

3. Press the right hand to the right and the left hand to the left, so that the palms are now facing each other. The thumb of the right hand should pass in front of the little finger of the left. Now press the palms together (as much as is possible for you), lift your elbows up, and stretch the fingers toward the ceiling.

4. Stay for 15 to 30 seconds, then unwind the legs and arms and stand in Tadasana again. Repeat for the same length of time with the arms and legs reversed.

Gomukhasana (Cow Face Pose)

Steps

1. Sit in Dandasana (Staff Pose), then bend your knees and put your feet on the floor. Slide your left foot under the right knee to the outside of the right hip. Then cross your right leg over the left, stacking the right knee on top of the left, and bring the right foot to the outside of the left hip. Try to bring the heels equidistant from the hips: with the right leg on top, you will have to tug the right heel in closer to the left hip. Sit evenly on the sitting bones.

2. Inhale and stretch your right arm straight out to the right, parallel to the floor. Rotate your arm inwardly; the thumb will turn first toward the floor, and then point toward the wall behind you, with the palm facing the ceiling. This movement will roll your right shoulder slightly up and forward, and round your upper back. With a full exhalation, sweep the arm behind your torso and tuck the forearm in the hollow of your lower back, parallel to your waist, with the right elbow against the right side of your torso. Roll the shoulder back and down, then work the forearm

up your back until it is parallel to your spine. The back of your hand will be between your shoulder blades. See that your right elbow does not slip away from the right side of your torso.

3. Now inhale and stretch your left arm straightforward, pointing toward the opposite wall, parallel to the floor. Turn the palm up and, with another inhalation, stretch the arm straight up toward the ceiling, palm turned back. Lift actively through your left arm, then with an exhalation, bend the elbow and reach down for the right hand. If possible, hook the right and left fingers.

4. Lift the left elbow toward the ceiling and, from the back armpit, descend the right elbow toward the floor. Firm your shoulder blades against your back ribs and lift your chest. Try to keep the left arm right beside the left side of your head.

5. Stay in this pose about 1 minute. Release the arms, uncross the legs, and repeat with the arms and legs reversed for the same length of time. Remember that whichever leg is on top, the same-side arm is lower.

Try to practice these poses every 20 minutes, holding the pose 30 to 60 seconds. If the area you are in seems a little tight don't worry you can practice the mountain pose or the eagle pose because they take the least amount of space. Remember, you need to take care of yourself because no one is going to do it for you and stress is the main cause most illnesses. Stress wears your body and leaves your body open for attack! So do those poses and relieve that stress.

25. Diagnosed with Cancer: What Is The Next Step?

Written by Theresa Ann Gill
A breast cancer survivor

Reflection

Whether they are good or bad, a life-changing situation often gives people a chance to grow, appreciate and learn what is important to them in their lives. I for one can describe my battle with cancer as a personal journey with myself. This time in my life allowed me to reflect on my relationships with others, it gave me time to make peace with people around me; I became more tolerant of my world as well as more spiritual. I found time in my life to mediate and maintain a healthy mind as well as body.
This was not necessarily a journey that I would have chosen for myself but because this was the journey that I had to pursue because of my illness. I vowed to do this with a positive attitude. I used my skills, strength and talents to venture on this journey with a hopeful outlook.

One of the first things I did was make a set of rules for myself to live by. Some may say that it was selfish but I always believed that if you do not love yourself with all your heart then you could not love another because you will not have the ability to understand how to do this. My rules to help me survive and cope are listed below. I hope they help you as much as they have helped me.

Terri Survival Rules

- o **Rule # 1 -** I will take care of myself the best way I know how. This will allow me to take care of my family because I will keep myself strong and healthy.
- o **Rule #2 - I** will also have people help me if I cannot do the tasks that I use to do.

- Rule #3 - I will accept the limitations of my strength during the time of my illness.
- **Rule** - I have the right to get angry and feel vulnerable but I will not feel sorry for myself.
- **Rule #5** - I will not let this curve ball in my life shatter hope, cripple love or conquer my Spirit.
- **Rule #6** - I will laugh everyday
- **Rule #7** - I will not take everything so seriously
- **Rule #8** I will remember that I am connected to every other person on the planet
- **Rule #9** I will give myself up to whatever the moment brings
- **Rule #10** - I will ask more than usual of myself

Your diagnosis

When you first hear that you have cancer, your initial response is will I die from it. Approximately 10 million Americans who are alive have a history of cancer. For many people cancer is an on-going health problem just like cholesterol, and heart disease. After your cancer treatments ends you will start feeling like your old self. You have to get regular check-ups this is very important in order to keep things in check.

The most important thing that you can do is focus on the living. Keep in mind that cancer is not always a death sentence. Many will go on to live a long and wonderful life. It is important to make the most out of each day that you have. Even though you may at times have feelings of fear, anxiety, guilt, anger and even denial it is important to have hope. This is the most important feeling of your life. It is also very important to talk about your feelings with others because this can relieve stress. If you have stress then this can prevent your body from fighting the disease as it should and lower your immune system even more.

Dealing with Stress

Some of the things that helped me deal with stress were exercising. Many of you may say I do not even exercise now how will I be able to do this while going through treatment. This goes back to Rule number 1. I will take care of myself the best way I know how. Exercise helps you relax and relives stress. I also did a lot of yoga and mediating which also combats stress. I did a lot of reading of various different types of books. I kept myself busy so that I would not have time to feel sorry for myself. That just would not accomplish anything. The main idea here is to find ways to control stress and not let stress control you.

Dealing with Pain

Treatment sucks. I am not going to lie. What I did every time I had to go for treatment was getting dressed up. My husband would take me to a wonderful lunch in a very nice restaurant because I knew that I would be sick for days later and food would taste like metal so I had a pre-treatment date. It made the inevitable tolerable. If you feel good going into the treatment then the outcome is not that hard to deal with. When I came home, I rested and in a couple of days, I was able to move on.

Other ways I dealt with pain and discomfort was getting a massage, imagery, such as thinking about a "happy place." Remember **Happy Gilmore**. Trust me it works. There is no reason for you to be bothered with pain and discomfort we are in the 21st century. If all else fails your doctor will prescribe you something. Remember you are the only person who can decide how much pain you feel. I personally do not like to deal with drugs unless I absolutely have to so I try all alternative methods first but remember this is something that you and your doctor can decide together.

Self-control

I am a person who likes to be in charge of my life. I have an A type personality. Naturally, when I was diagnosed with cancer this made me feel as if my life was out of control. Breast cancer was not something I was familiar dealing with. This was a completely new experience. One that I was not emotionally prepared to deal with at the time. I created coping strategies. They helped me get through breast cancer. Now I would like to share them with you.

Terri's Coping Strategies

- o The way I dealt with this was to learn as much as I could about the cancer I had.
- o I stayed busy; I continued pursing my education I was in college at the time.
- o I tried to keep my life as normal as possible.
- o I did not feel sorry for myself.
- o If I remained in control then the people around me modeled my behavior.
- o By staying positive in my thoughts and actions, others did the same.
- o I was able to keep people informed because I learned all that was needed to about my illness and my course of action to recover.
- o Remember to "Turn your face to the sun and the shadows fall behind you." – *Maori Proverb*

Another way to keep self-control is surround yourself with positive people. Many people feel guilty about their illness with cancer. You feel that you will be a burden to others. You may even become jealous of people who are healthy. This is normal in the beginning but you have to realize that guilt will not change anything. Cancer can just happen. It is no ones fault. We all have a cancer gene in our body that lies dormant and for some it wakes up one day and grows out of control. This is a nonprofessional's way to look at it. Life threw you a curve ball and you were not ready to send it out of the park. If you cannot realize this then seek out counseling and support groups that can help you deal with this. The most important thing is that you start to move forward.

Long Term Outlook

Keep a journal and write down your feelings. One thing that works is everyday make a commitment to write down five things in your life you are happy about. I am serious. This will allow you to look for reasons of hope. Plan your days with little things that you want to do. Make goals for yourself. You can and will lead an active life even during your treatment. Remember however dark it may seem a new day will dawn tomorrow.

Dealing with telling your Children about Cancer

I had three young children ages 13, 11, and 9. I waited to tell them until I had all the facts. I made sure that I was able to deal with whatever emotions they were going to have. The only way to do this is to be able to deal with this yourself. I first let their teachers know about my diagnosis so that they can monitor any unusual behavior they might see in my children. I also made sure that I had booked my appointment for my surgery so that I would be able to be honest with my children about what was going to take place and how long I would be staying in the hospital as well what kind of treatments I would be having in the future. I gave my children the opportunity to ask questions and express their feelings. I also used terms that they could understand and when I told them I already had in place friends who would help with any carpooling that I needed so that my children's activities could continue and I ensured my children that their lives would continue as normal.

In the beginning, my children were scared and confused but over time, they realized that things were going to be okay and although I was tired a lot more, we spent quality time together watching movies, reading stories

The most important thing here is to be honest and open with your children, family and friends about your cancer as well as any feelings that arise and handle each issue in the early stages. This will help with any change that arises in each of their lives.

Do Not Deal With Cancer Alone

It is important to share your thoughts and feelings about cancer with someone. If for some reason you do not have a support group within your immediate friends and family then it is important to turn to your church, synagogue, hospital or local library to find a group or counselor that will be able to provide you with the support you need.

Remember, never doubt that a small group of thoughtful, empathetic, caring and committed people can change the world. It is important to have support during these tough times. Have people by your side to support and comfort you means a lot.

Keep your hopes high and your smiles wide in life, you only have one!

About Juicing

I mentioned earlier that when you go for chemo you feel terrible. Food tastes like metal. In order to keep your strength up I have found that juicing helped. It gave you the vitamins that you needed, but were not allowed to take in pill form and satisfied your hunger without having to deal with long drawn out meals that were hard to keep down.

Many books have been written on how uncooked foods or "raw foods" help with diseases such as cancer. They help the immune system heal itself. In actuality, many fruits and vegetables have nutrients that kill cancer cells and or stop the spread of cancer. The definition of raw food means food eaten without cooking. All I used to create these juices were a food processor and juicer. Both they sell at a reasonable cost in stores light Target, Wal-Mart, Sears, to name a few.

To give you a little background on the subject I will say that cooking food destroys 100% of all enzymes in a food. I am not suggesting throwing out your pots and pans but instead to incorporate raw foods into your diet. I am also suggesting that cooking food places a great burden on our body and does not allow you to get as many nutrients out of the food. These nutrients are vital especially when fighting a disease like cancer.

Before you stop eating all cook foods I will also say that some nutrients are made more readily available by cooking, I am just suggesting that overall it is better to eat vegetables and fruits raw instead of cooked

Here is a list of the RAW vegetables you should be juicing: Carrots, broccoli, red beets, and beet top as well, peppers, cabbage, green asparagus and the spice turmeric.

In addition, a note to everyone who juices beets your urine can possible turn red do not be alarmed it doe not mean you have blood in your urine.

Fruits are also important to juice as well, you should be incorporating these into your diet as well: purple grapes with skins and seeds the whole thing can be put in the juicer, red raspberries, black berries, strawberries, peaces, apricots blueberries, pineapples and tomatoes.

Last but not least is wheatgrass, this can be purchased both frozen at a health food store and popped into your juice or you can buy it buy the shot at a place like Mrs. Greens.

Wheatgrass is immediately absorbed in the bloodstream and gives you an immediate boost of energy. This is something you lack when going through chemo. It also has been proven to build red blood cells quickly after you ingest it. Wheatgrass has been known to normalize high blood pressure and stimulate healthy tissue cell growth.

The Recipes

The following are mixes you can put into your juicer and blend away.

🔸 Carrot/Apple Juice
6 carrots
2 apples

Wash and peel the carrots. Unless you use organic fruits and vegetables then just wash. Wash everything else, and cut up into sections if needed. Juice everything and enjoy

↲ Beet Special

2-3 carrots
½ beet

Wash and peel the carrots. Wash everything else, and cut up into sections if needed. Juice everything and enjoy

↲ Pineapple Delight

Pineapple (skin & all) ☐unscrew top and throw away
2 oranges
1 grapefruit

Wash everything cut into slices. Juice everything and enjoy.

↲ Keep the Doctor Away

2 apples
1 pear

Wash everything cut into slices. Juice everything and enjoy.

↲ Veggie Cocktail

Handful of spinach
6 carrots

Wash everything cut into slices. Juice everything and enjoy.

♦ Thirst Quencher

2 apples
1 large bunch of grapes
1 slice lemon with peel

Wash everything cut into slices. Juice everything and enjoy.

♦ Detox

4 carrots
½ cucumber
1 beet

Wash everything cut into slices. Juice everything and enjoy.

♦ Energizer Bunny

Handful of parsley
3 carrots
2 celery stalks
2 cloves of garlic
Cantaloupe Juice

Cut into strips and juice (rind and all)

♦ Veggie Juice

4 medium potatoes
4 medium carrots
1 stalk of broccoli
6 brussel sprouts
1 cucumber

Wash all of the vegetables and cut into sections. Juice the potatoes with their skin on and set aside. Juice the carrots and set aside. Juice the rest of the ingredients together. Combine all of the juice, stir and enjoy!

✦ Apple Carrot Juice

2 apples
6 carrots

Wash everything, peel the carrots and cut into sections where needed. Juice everything.

✦ Carrot Anise Juice

8 carrots
2 anise stalks
3-4 celery stalks
2 apples

Wash and peel the carrots. Wash everything else, and cut up into sections if needed. Juice everything and enjoy

✦ Carrot, Celery, Cabbage Combo #1

3-4 Carrots
1-2 Celery stalks
Small wedge cabbage

Wash all vegetables and juice.

✦ Carrot, Celery, Cabbage Combo

2 carrots
2 cucumbers
2 stalks of celery
A piece of ginger
A handful of parsley
A piece of apple or citrus fruit

Wash all vegetables and juice.

✦ Carrot Combination

2 1/2 lbs. carrots
1 beet with greens
1 stalk celery
1 large handful spinach
1 large handful parsley
1 green pepper
1 clove garlic
1 slice ginger

Wash and peel carrots. Clean and slice beet into thin wedges. Wash and dry spinach leaves and parsley. Juice half of the carrots and beet. Add the remaining ingredients by using the remaining carrots and push them through the juicer. Complete by juicing carrots.

✦ Carrot Glow

4 carrots
1 beet with greens
5 - 6 leaves of Romaine or other leaf lettuce
3 - 4 leaves of spinach

Wash and peel the carrots. Clean and cut beet into sections, and wash & dry lettuce and spinach leaves. Juice half of the carrots, and the beet, and then use the remaining carrots to help push the lettuce and spinach through the juicer.

✦ Carrot Grass

3 carrots
2-3 inch round of wheatgrass

Wash and peel the carrots, then juice with the wheatgrass. You can add ¼ cup of water if it is too strong.

↓ Carrot Parsley Juice
3 carrots
50 g (2 oz) parsley

Peel the carrots and wash the parsley, then juice.

↓ Carrot Strawberry Juice
4-6 Carrots
6 Strawberries

Wash and peel the carrots. Wash the strawberries. Alternate the carrots and strawberries through the juicer.

↓ Vibrant Carrot Juice
1 small beet
1 pear
1 apple
Small piece of ginger 2 inches salsify root
4 celery stalks
10-12 carrots
1 small parsnip

Wash everything and cut into smaller sections. Juice and be surprised at the wonderful colors before you mix it all together.

↓ Garden Tonic
Handful of spinach
3 stalks of celery
1 large tomato
1 cherry tomato (garnish)

Bunch up the spinach and juice with the celery the set aside. Juice the asparagus with the tomato. Combine the two mixtures, stir and garnish with the cherry tomato

♦ Hot Pepper Juice

1 large carrot
1 sweet apple
1 tomato
½ cucumber
½ bell pepper
1 stalk celery
1 zucchini
2 or 3 pepperoncinis

Juice the carrot, apple and tomato together and set aside. Next juice the cucumber, bell pepper, celery, zucchini and pepperoncinis. Combine the two mixtures, stir and drink immediately.

♦ Unbelievable Juice

1 cucumber
1 small beet
½ rhubarb stalk
1 apple
8 carrots
1 small purple top turnip
5 celery stalks

Wash, peel and cut into sections where needed. Juice everything separately and combine.

♦ Pineapple Carrot Juice

3-4 large carrots
4-6 rounds of pineapple

Wash and peel the carrots. Put the carrots through the juicer first, and then the pineapple. Serve over ice.

↓ Purification tablet

3 carrots
1/2 cucumber
1/2 beet with the greens

Wash everything. Cut the cucumber into quarters and strips. Cut the beet into sections. Process it all in your juicer.

↓ Relaxation Juice

4 carrots
1/2 cucumber

Wash everything, cut into sections, and process in your juicer.

↓ Rejuvenation Juice

8 large carrots
1/2 large beet
1/2 turnip
1/2 parsnip
5 celery stalks
1/4 rutabaga
1/8 head red cabbage.
5 radishes
1 large apple
1 cup cranberries

Wash everything, peel where needed and cut into sections where needed. Juice together in your juicer, mix and enjoy!

⚜ Battle Juice
6 carrots
2 stalks of celery
Handful of parsley
2 cloves of garlic

Wash everything and cut the carrots and celery into sections. Begin juicing with the garlic and then juice everything else

⚜ Aromatic Mix
3-4 carrots
1 stalk celery
1/2 cup chopped parsley
1/2 cup chopped spinach, packed

Wash everything, peel the carrots and dry the leafy greens. Juice them together in the order given.

⚜ Just Green
2 stalks of celery
3 asparagus
4 large spinach leaves
1 half cup parsley
2-3 inch round of wheatgrass

Wash greens thoroughly, cut up celery and juice. You can dilute this juice with ¼ cup of water if it is too strong.

⚜ Fiery Tomato Juice
6 tomatoes
1 cup beet leaves, chopped
1 slice lemon

Cut the tomatoes up into sections and juice everything in the order given in the ingredient list.

✦ Spinach Power

5 carrots
6 spinach leaves
4 lettuce leaves
1/4 turnip
4 sprigs of parsley

Wash everything, peel the carrots, cut into sections where needed, and juice.

✦ Stomach Soother

½ head cabbage
1 beet (with greens)
2 large kiwis

Wash the cabbage and beet and then cut everything into sections that can fit in your juice. Juice together.

✦ Zesty Carrot Juice

1 beet with greens
1 stalk celery
1 large handful spinach
1 large handful parsley
1 green pepper
1 clove garlic
1 slice ginger
2 ½ pounds carrots

Wash and peel carrots. Wash and cut beets into sections, and wash & dry parsley and spinach leaves. Juice half of the carrots, and the beet, and then use the remaining carrots to help push the rest through the juicer.

Sweet Carrot Juice

5 Carrots
1 Apple
1/2 Beet

Wash fruit and vegetables. Cut the apple and beet into sections and juice everything

Swiss Chard Celery Juice

4 carrots
2 apples
½ cucumber
1 stalk celery
1 small bunch Swiss chard

Separately juice the carrots, apples, cucumber, celery and Swiss chard. Once you are finished juicing, combine all of the juices, stir and drink immediately.

Tingling Cabbage Juice

3 medium carrots
¼ heard of cabbage
1 stalk of celery
5 pitted cherries

Wash everything and slice the head of cabbage into smaller pieces. Juice the carrots and set aside. Juice the cabbage and celery together and put aside. Juice the cherries and combine all of the fresh juices together.

Yummy Green Juice

2 green apples
4 stalks celery
8 stalks bok choy
¼ pound spinach
1 bunch parsley
Recipe continued on next page...

110

Wash everything and cut into sections where needed. Juice the apples and set aside. Juice everything else together and combine with the apple juice when done. Stir and enjoy

✦ Tomato Light

4 ripe tomatoes
1 cup green lettuce, packed

Cut the tomatoes up into sections and juice everything in the order given in the ingredient list.

✦ Tomato Burst

6 carrots
2 tomatoes
1 stalk celery

Cut the tomatoes up into sections and juice everything in the order given in the ingredient list.

✦ Veggie Delicious

2 large carrots
3 stalks celery
1/2 cup parsley
4 large spinach leaves
1/2 beet root
1/2 cup alfalfa sprouts

Wash veggies thoroughly and cut into sections where needed. Juice everything and enjoy!

Be creative, try some new combinations. They are all wonderful. Savor big joys and small pleasures.

Sections 5

Stories & Poetry about Breast Cancer

26. Stories & Poetry about Breast Cancer

You're a Survivor

Written by Jill Eisnaugle
Author of Coastal Whispers & Under Amber Skies

In one single moment, the world you knew changed
Each second of glory had been rearranged
The sky above, once filled with wonder and light
Became dark and lonely, yet you chose to fight
With your friends and family, there by your side
You mustered the courage to battle in stride
With faith as a beacon to guide you along
You began a journey, which would make you strong.

At times, you knew conflict; therefore, tears were shed
Yet, you remained focused on the goal, ahead
To overcome cancer, one mile at a time
Despite every mountain you were asked to climb
You always found comfort in the countless prayers
Issued in your name, sent to God's golden stairs
And thus, every morning, you rose for the day
Ready for each challenge that could come your way.

In one single moment, the life you knew ceased
Yet, you were determined to conquer the beast
Although, you had cancer, afflicting your breast
You realized your life was incredibly blessed
So, armed with your courage and your flare for life
You rose from the valley of sadness and strife
To defeat your illness, by taking a stand
Now, you're a survivor, just as God had planned!

Optimism

Optimistic people bring a sense of hope into world. Encouraging people bring a new meaning to life. They help you see past the clouds on a glooming day. They bring sunlight everyday

Life's Obstacles

Life comes with obstacles. Obstacles that must be pursued. No matter how rough the obstacle. You will succeed if you focus on the positive.

A New Beginning

There comes a time when the meaning of life begins to make sense,
At first we may not understand why things happen the way they do,
The sky at first may look dark,
The path one needs to walk down may be hard to see,
Remember the stars are the brightest when the nights seem the darkest
Look up at the stars and make a wish
One wish
Never let the fact that you have breast cancer control your destiny,
Move forward,
Never move backwards
Plan a positive, fulfilling future,
Never let your tragedy control your mind, body and soul,
Never give up,
Be in control,
Accept yourself,
Accept your disease,
Love yourself now and forever,
Developing breast cancer
Makes you feel barricaded against a corner
Giving up is not an option,
The present is now,
Today is a new day,
If you stay down life will pass you by,
Therefore, each time you fall
Help yourself get up,
Fight the battle
Win your battle,
To win the battle all you need to do is try,
Winning the battle is teaching yourself how to live a healthy productive life,
Helping you cope,
Life may not always be what you planned it to be,
The road you lead may have some u-turns involved,
Do not fear,

For change can be good,
Follow the path that was destined for you,
The sun is now shinning,
You can now see your path
There is a plan, a destiny that awaits you,
Do not question your destiny,
Do not ask questions such as "why me?"
Follow life's journey the one that has been planned for you.
Do not be afraid,
Take one day at a time,
Be proud of who you are,
Walk with courage and your head up high,
Believe in yourself,
Focus on the positive,
For the footsteps imbedded in ground of your new path will
become the solid foundation to you future.

Believe In Your Heart

I woke up one night in the hours of darkness,
I sat up straight in my bed to find a shimmering light in my
closet,
But their where no lights on in the room,
I got up and went slowly toward the closet,
To find a pair of gold wings,
An angel was standing by my side,
"What do I do with these gold wings?" I asked the angel
"Put the wings on my child." Answered the angel
I put the wings on flew to a place that had many stars,
The angel then appeared and said, "Follow your heart, your
goals and your dreams."
Only you know what is right for you
Anything is possible
Miracles do come true,
Hope and dreams are a reality if let them be,
Life can be wonderful if you let it be,
The world is at your feet
Therefore, there is no time waste,
Start flying to the stars,
The bright star in the sky created especially for you,
Therefore, there is no time to lose go find your bright star,
When you find it, open the magic door
Out will come gifts,
Waiting for you to explore,
So believe in your dreams
Follow your heart
Your world can be a happier place as long as you believe.

27. Breast Cancer: Resources

Organizations

American Cancer Society

Phone: 1-800-ACS-2345 (1-800-227-2345)

Web Address: http://www.cancer.org

The American Cancer Society conducts educational programs and offers many services to people with cancer and their families. Staff at the toll-free number has information about services and activities in local areas and can provide referrals to local ACS divisions.

National Alliance of Breast Cancer Organizations (NABCO)

Phone: (212) 889-0606

E-mail: NABCOinfo@aol.com

Web Address: http://www.nabco.org/

Founded in 1986, the National Alliance of Breast Cancer Organizations (NABCO) is the leading nonprofit information and education resource on breast cancer. It is a network of with 400 member organizations and agencies in the United States that provides education to the public, as well as information, resources, and referrals to medical professionals and their organizations. All NABCO services are offered free of charge. NABCO also works on the community, state, and federal levels for regulatory change and legislation to benefit those with cancer, survivors, and those at risk.

National Breast Cancer Coalition (NBCC)

1101 17th Street, N.W.

Suite 1300

Washington, DC 20036

Information about NBCC continued on the next page...

Phone:	1-800-622-2838
	(202) 296-7477
Fax:	(202) 265-6854
Web Address:	http://www.natlbcc.org

The National Breast Cancer Coalition (NBCC) is a grassroots advocacy organization dedicated to fighting breast cancer.

National Cancer Institute (NCI)

NCI Publications Office

6116 Executive Boulevard, MSC8322

Suite 3036A

Bethesda, MD 20892-8322

Phone:	1-800-4-CANCER (1-800-422-6237)
Web Address:	http://www.cancer.gov

The National Cancer Institute is a government agency that provides up-to-date information about cancer and its prevention, detection, treatment, and supportive care to people with cancer and their families. NCI information is also available to doctors, nurses, and other health professionals. NCI provides the latest information about clinical trials. The Cancer Information Service, a service of NCI, has trained staff members available to answer questions and send free publications. Spanish-speaking staff is also available.

Y-ME National Breast Cancer Organization, Inc.

212 West Van Buren Street

Suite 1000

Chicago, IL 60607-3903

Phone:	1-800-221-2141 (English)

```
                    1-800-986-9505 (Spanish)
Fax:                (312) 986-8338
Web Address:        http://www.y-me.org
```

Y-ME National Breast Cancer Organization has a commitment
to provide support to anyone who has been touched by breast
cancer. Two breast cancer patients founded Y-ME in 1978,
when they realized that women who had experienced breast
cancer could best meet their needs for information and
support. Since the beginning, Y-ME has served women with
breast cancer and their families and friends through their
national hotline, open-door groups, early detection workshops,
and local chapters. The hotline provides interpreters in many
languages.

Susan G. Komen Foundation

The Susan G. Komen Foundation supports research and
community-based outreach programs related to breast cancer.
This link will take you to the web site.

National Breast Cancer Foundation

The National Breast Cancer Foundation works to increase
breast cancer awareness and to provide mammograms for
those in need. This link will take you to its web site.

National Cancer Institute

The National Cancer Institute is part of the U.S. National
Institutes of Health (NIH). This link will take you to the web
site.

Young Survival Coalition

This international nonprofit group is dedicated to the concerns
and issues of young women with breast cancer. This link will
take you to its web site.

Intercultural Cancer Council

The Intercultural Cancer Council promotes cancer research, policies, programs, and partnerships in racial and ethnic minorities as well as medically underserved groups in the U.S. This link will take you to the web site.

28. Breast Cancer Glossary

A

Ablative therapy: Treatment that involves the removal or destruction of the function of an organ, as in the surgical removal of the ovaries or the administration of some types of chemotherapy that causes the ovaries to stop functioning.

Abscess: A closed pocket of tissue containing pus (a creamy, thick, pale yellow or yellow-green fluid that comes from dead tissue); most commonly caused by a bacterial infection.

Accessory breast tissue: An uncommon condition in which additional breast tissue is found in the axillary (underarm) area. Women with this condition often require special mammography views.

Acini: Another term for the lobules of the breast. Lobules are milk-producing glands.

Adenocarcinoma: Cancer that originates in the glandular tissue, such as in the ducts or lobules of the breast.

Adenoma: A benign growth originating in the glandular tissue of the breast that can compress adjacent tissue as it grows in size. (See also fibroadenoma).

Adjuvant therapy: Additional treatment that is added to increase the effectiveness of a primary therapy. Common types of adjuvant therapy include: hormonal therapy, chemotherapy, or radiation added after surgery to increase the chances of curing the disease or keeping it in check.

Adrenal gland: One adrenal gland is located near each kidney. Their main function is to produce hormones that regulate metabolism and control fluid balance and blood pressure. Adrenal glands also produce small amounts of "male" hormones (androgens) and "female" hormones (estrogens and progesterone).

Advanced cancer: A stage of cancer in which the disease has spread from the primary site to other parts of the body. When the cancer has spread only to the surrounding areas, it is called locally advanced. If it has spread further by traveling through the bloodstream, it is called distantly advanced or metastatic.

Alopecia: Hair loss. Temporary alopecia often occurs because of chemotherapy or less commonly, when radiation therapy is administered to the head.

Alternative treatment: See therapy.

Anastrozole (brand name, Arimidex): See Arimidex.

Androgen: A male sex hormone. Androgens may be used to treat recurrent breast cancer. Their purpose is to oppose the activity of estrogen, thereby slowing growth of the cancer.

Anesthesia: The loss of feeling or sensation because of drugs or gases. General anesthesia causes loss of consciousness ("puts you to sleep"). Local or regional anesthesia causes loss of feeling only to a specified area.

Aneuploid: An abnormal number of chromosomes; a characteristic of cancer. (See also ploidy).

Antibiotic: Chemical substances produced by living organisms or synthesized (created) in laboratories, for killing other organisms that cause disease. Some cancer therapies interfere with the body's ability to fight off infection (they suppress the immune system), so antibiotics may be needed along with the cancer treatment to prevent or treat infections.

Antibody: An immune system protein in the blood that defends against invading foreign agents, such as bacteria. Invading agents contain certain chemical substances called antigens. Each antibody works against a specific antigen. (See also antigen).

Antiemetic: Also spelled antemetic. A drug used to control nausea and vomiting (emesis), which are common side effects of chemotherapy. Antiemetic drugs can be used before, during, or after chemotherapy. Granisetron and ondansetron are examples of antiemetic drugs.

Antiestrogen: A substance that blocks the effects of the hormone estrogen on tumors (for example, the drug tamoxifen). Antiestrogens are used to treat breast cancers that depend on estrogen for growth.

Antigen: A chemical substance that stimulates an immune system response. This reaction often involves production of antibodies. For example, the immune system's response to antigens that are part of bacteria and viruses helps people resist infections. Cancer cells have certain antigens that can be detected by laboratory tests, and are important in cancer diagnosis and in monitoring response to treatment. Other cancer cell antigens play a role in immune reactions that may help the body's resistance against cancer.

Antimetabolites: Substances that interfere with the body's chemical processes, such as creating proteins, DNA, and other chemicals needed for cell growth and reproduction. In treating cancer, antimetabolite drugs interfere with DNA production, which in turn prevents cell division and growth of tumors. (See also DNA).

Areola: The dark pigmented area that encircles the nipple.

Arimidex (generic name, anastrozole): A drug sometimes used to treat advanced breast cancer in post-menopausal women who have not responded well to treatment with the drug tamoxifen.

Aromasin: Brand name of exemestane. Drug used to treat metastatic breast cancer in post-menopausal women. Works by binding to the body's aromastase enzyme, an enzyme responsible for producing the hormone, estrogen.

Aspiration: Removal of tissue or fluid from a lump or cyst with a needle and syringe. (See also needle aspiration).

Asymmetry: An area that is not found to be identical in both breasts (such as tissue density). It is often a normal variant but can also be a sign of an abnormal growth.

Asymmetrical: Not proportional or the same. It is normal for women to have slightly asymmetrical breasts.

Asymptomatic: To be without noticeable symptoms of disease (literally "not symptomatic" or no symptoms of the disease). Many cancers can develop and grow without producing symptoms, especially in the early stages. Screening tests, such as mammography, try to discover developing cancers at the asymptomatic stage, when the chances for cure are usually highest. (See also screening).

Atypical: Literally, "not typical." Exhibits unusual characteristics. For example, atypical hyperplasia is a dangerous increase in the number of breast cells; a sign that breast cancer may develop.

Augmentation mammoplasty: Surgery to increase the size of the breast(s). Also called breast augmentation surgery.

Autologous: Using one's own tissue. An autologous reconstruction uses the patient's own tissue to reconstruct the breast.

Axilla: The armpit. (See also axillary dissection).

Axillary node dissection: A surgical procedure in which the lymph nodes in the armpit (axillary nodes) are removed and examined to find out if breast cancer has spread to those nodes and to remove any cancerous lymph nodes.

B

Benign: Not cancerous; not malignant. The main types of benign breast problems are fibroadenomas and fibrocystic change. (See also fibroadenoma, fibrocystic change).

Bilateral: Affecting both sides of the body; for example, bilateral breast cancer is cancer occurring in both breasts at the same time (synchronous) or at different times (metachronous).

Biologic response modifiers: Substances that boost the body's immune system to fight against cancer. (See also interferon).

Biological therapy: Treatment to restore the ability of the immune system to fight infection or other diseases.

Biopsy: A procedure in which tissue samples are removed from the body for examination of their appearance under a microscope to find out whether cancer or other abnormal cells are present. A biopsy can be done with a needle or by surgery.

Blood count: The number of red blood cells, white blood cells, and platelets in a sample of blood. Also called complete blood count (CBC).

Bone densitometry: Exam used to measure a patient's bone mineral density of various parts of the body, such as the spine, hip, heel, or wrist. The exam is useful in determining whether a patient has osteoporosis.

Bone marrow transplant: A complex treatment that may be used when breast cancer is advanced or has recurred. The bone marrow transplant makes it possible to use very high doses of chemotherapy that would otherwise be impossible. Autologous bone marrow transplant means that the patient's own bone marrow is used. An allogeneic bone marrow transplant uses marrow from a donor whose tissue type closely matches the patient's. A portion of the patient's or donor's bone marrow is withdrawn, cleansed, treated, and stored. The patient is then given high doses of chemotherapy that kill the cancer cells but also destroy the remaining bone marrow, thus robbing the body of its natural ability to fight infection. The cleansed and stored marrow is given by transfusion (transplanted) to rescue the patient's immune defenses. Although this method has been widely reported by the media, and it has given good results in many people, it has not been scientifically proven to be more effective than conventional therapies in treating breast cancer. It is a risky procedure that involves a lengthy and expensive hospital stay that may not be covered by the patient's health insurance. The best place to have a bone marrow transplant is at a comprehensive cancer center or other facility that has the technical skill and experience to perform it safely.

Bone scan: A nuclear medicine imaging method that gives important information about the bones, including the location of cancer that may have spread to the bones. It can be done as an outpatient procedure and is usually painless, except for the needle stick when a low-dose radioactive substance is injected into a vein. Images are taken to see where the radioactivity accumulates, indicating an abnormality.

Bone (skeletal) survey: X-ray imaging of the entire skeleton.

Bracytherapy: A technique that involves placing radioactive substances directly into body tissue next to the cancer. Bracytherapy is currently being developed to use on breast cancer patients. Also called internal radiation.

Brain scan: A nuclear medicine imaging method used to find abnormalities in the brain, including brain cancer and cancer that has spread to the brain from other places in the body. This procedure can be done in an outpatient clinic. It is painless, except for the needle stick when a radioactive substance is injected into a vein. The images taken will show where radioactivity accumulates, indicating an abnormality.

BRCA1: Breast Cancer Gene 1. A gene which, when damaged (mutated), places a woman at greater risk of developing breast and/or ovarian cancer, compared with women who do not have the mutation. In a woman with a BRCA1 mutation, the estimated lifetime risk of developing breast cancer is about 50% compared with about 12% in the general population. A person who has this mutated gene has a 50% chance of passing on the gene to each of her children. A genetic test is available, but it is recommended only for women who are known to be at risk because several women in their family have had breast or ovarian cancer at an early age (before menopause). Any women considering the test should consider receiving genetic counseling.

BRCA2: Breast Cancer Gene 2. A gene which, when damaged or mutated, puts the carrier at a higher risk for developing breast cancer and/or ovarian cancer than the general population. In a woman with a BRCA2 mutation, the estimated lifetime risk of developing breast cancer is 50% - 60%. BRCA2 and BRCA1 together account for about 80% of the breast cancers that occur in women with strong family histories of the disease. BRCA2 is also thought to raise the risk for breast cancer in men. A genetic test for BRCA2 is available but is only recommended for women or men with strong family histories of breast or ovarian cancer. Any women considering the test should consider receiving genetic counseling.

Breast augmentation surgery: Surgery to increase the size of the breast(s). Also called augmentation mammoplasty.

Breast biopsy: The removal of breast cells for pathological examination. A breast biopsy is performed to determine whether a suspicious area of the breast is cancerous or benign.

Breast cancer: Cancer that originates in the breast. The main types of breast cancer are ductal carcinoma in situ, invasive ductal carcinoma, invasive lobular carcinoma, medullary carcinoma, and Paget's disease of the nipple. Lobular carcinoma in situ (LCIS) is sometimes considered to be a type of breast cancer, but most breast specialists feel LCIS is a marker for increased breast cancer risk, and not a true cancer. (See definitions of these terms).

Breast compression: The flattening of the breast so that the maximum amount of tissue can be imaged and examined during mammography.

Breast conservation therapy: Also called lumpectomy; the surgical removal of a cancerous breast lump and a small amount of non-cancerous tissue around the lump, without removing any other part of the breast. The method may or may not require an axillary dissection. Breast conservation therapy is usually followed by at least six weeks of radiation. (See also lumpectomy and radiation therapy).

Breast density: Describes breast tissue that has many glands close together. Density shows up as a white area on a mammogram film. Though fairly common (especially in younger women), dense breasts may make microcalcifications and many other masses difficult to detect.

Breast expander: A device used to stretch the remaining breast skin after a mastectomy. A breast expander is similar to a balloon, and the surgeon will fill the expander with salt-water solution periodically (usually once a week). The expansion process typically takes three to four months. After the skin is sufficiently stretched, the surgeon will replace the expander with a permanent breast implant. Also called tissue expander.

Breast-feeding: Giving a baby milk from the breast. Also called suckling or nursing.

Breast implant: A manufactured sac that is filled with silicone gel (a synthetic material) or saline (sterile saltwater). The sac is surgically inserted to increase breast size or restore the contour of a breast after mastectomy (breast removal). Because of concern about possible (but unproven) side effects of silicone, silicone implants are presently available only to women who agree to participate in a clinical trial in which side effects are carefully monitored.

Breast lift surgery: See mastoplexy.

Breast pain: Cyclic or non-cyclic pain in the breast or in the axilla (underarm) region of the body. Approximately 15% of women with breast pain require treatment. Breast pain is not usually (but can be) associated with breast cancer. Also called mastalgia.

Breast prosthesis: An external breast form. Some women wear prostheses after mastectomy (breast removal). Many prostheses resemble the body's own weight and touch.

Breast reconstruction: Surgery that rebuilds the breast contour after mastectomy. A breast implant or the woman's own tissue provides the contour. If desired, the nipple and areola may also be re-created. Reconstruction can usually be done at the time of mastectomy or any time later. (See also mammoplasty).

Breast reduction surgery: Surgery to reduce the size of the breast(s). Also called reduction mammoplasty.

Breast repositioning: See mastoplexy.

Breast self-examination (BSE): A technique of checking one's own breasts for lumps or suspicious changes. The method is recommended for all women over age 20, to be done once a month. It is recommended that pre-menopausal women perform BSE the week after menstruation when the breasts are typically least tender.

Breast specialist: A term describing health care professionals who have a dedicated interest in breast health. While they may acquire specialized knowledge in this area, medical licensing boards do not certify a specialty in breast care.

C

Cachexia: General lack of nutrition or wasting that occurs in the course of some cancer cases.

Calcifications: Small calcium deposits within the breast, singly or in clusters, that are usually found by mammography. These are also called microcalcifications and macrocalcifications. They are a sign of change within the breast that may be monitored by additional, periodic mammograms, or by immediate or delayed biopsy. They may be caused by benign (non-cancerous) breast conditions or by breast cancer.

Cancer: A general term for more than 100 diseases in which malignant (cancerous) cells develop. Some exist quietly within the body for years without causing a problem. Others are aggressive, rapidly forming tumors that may invade and destroy surrounding tissue and travel through the lymph system or bloodstream to distant areas of the body.

Cancer care team: The group of health care professionals who cooperate in the diagnosis, treatment, after-care, and counseling of people with cancer. The breast cancer care team may include any or all of the following and others: primary care physician and/or gynecologist, pathologist, oncology specialists (medical oncologist, radiation oncologist), surgeon, nurse, oncology nurse specialist, oncology social worker. Whether the team is linked formally or informally, there is usually one person who takes the job of "referee." (See also case manager).

Cancer cell: A cell that divides and reproduces abnormally and can spread throughout the body. (See also metastasis).

Cancer-related checkup: A routine health examination for cancer in persons without obvious signs or symptoms of cancer. The goal of the cancer-related check-up is to find the disease, if it exists, at an early stage, when chances for cure are greatest. Clinical breast examinations, Pap smears, and skin examinations are examples of methods used in cancer-related check-ups. (See also detection, screening).

Capecitabine: Brand name, Xeloda. Drug used to treat metastatic breast cancer in patients who have not responded well to chemotherapy that included Taxol (generic name, paclitaxel) and an anthracycline (such as Adriamycin or doxorubicin). Capecitabine works by converting to a substance called 5-fluorouracil in the body. In some patients, capecitabine helps shrink tumor size by killing cancer cells.

Capsule formation: Scar tissue that may form around a breast (or other type of) implant as the body reacts to the foreign object. Sometimes called a contracture.

Carcinogen: Any substance that causes cancer or helps cancer to grow. For example, tobacco smoke contains many carcinogens that have been proven to dramatically increase the risk of lung cancer.

Carcinoma: A malignant (cancerous) tumor that begins in the lining layer (epithelial cells) of organs. At least 80% of all cancers are carcinomas, and almost all breast cancers are carcinomas.

Carcinoma in situ: An early stage of cancer, in which the tumor is still only in the structures of the organ where it first developed, and the disease has not invaded other parts of the organ or spread (metastasized). Most in situ carcinomas are highly curable.

Case manager: The member of a cancer care team—usually a nurse or oncology nurse specialist—who coordinates the patient's care throughout diagnosis, treatment, and recovery. The case manager is a new concept that provides a guide through the complex system of health care by helping cut through red tape, getting responses to questions, managing crises, and connecting the patient and family to needed resources.

Catheter: A thin tube through which fluids can enter and leave the body.

CT scan (CAT scan): See computed tomography.

Cell: The basic unit of all living organisms. Organs are clusters of cells that have developed specialized tasks. Cells replace themselves by splitting and forming new cells (mitosis). The processes that control formation of new cells and death of old cells are disrupted in cancer.

Chemoprevention: Prevention or reversal of disease using drugs, chemicals, vitamins, or minerals. While this idea is not currently widely used, it is a very promising area of study. The Breast Cancer Prevention Trial has shown that the drug tamoxifen can prevent some cases of breast cancer among women with high risk of this disease. However, the drug has some serious side effects.

Chemotherapy: Treatment with drugs to destroy cancer cells. Chemotherapy is often used in addition to surgery or radiation to treat cancer when metastasis (spread) is proven or suspected, when the cancer has come back (recurred), or when there is a strong likelihood that the cancer could recur. (See also adjuvant therapy).

Chest wall invasion: The growth of breast cancer into the pectoralis (chest wall) muscle; typically occurs with larger advanced cancers or with smaller cancers initially located near the pectoralis muscle.

Chromosome: A DNA molecule that contains genes arranged end-to-end. In humans and plants, chromosomes are located in the cell's nucleus (center).

Clear margins: Pathological term used to describe an adequate amount of normal tissue that is surgically removed along with the breast cancer.

Cleavage view: Also called "valley view," it is a mammogram view of the most medial portions of the breasts. This is the portion of breast tissue "in the valley" between the two breasts.

Clinical breast examination (CBE): A physical examination of the breast conducted by a health care professional such as a physician, physician assistant, nurse or nurse practitioner. The purpose of CBE is to detect lumps or suspicious breast changes that may warrant further attention.

Clinical trial: An organized research study conducted with people or animals to find new methods to prevent, detect, diagnose, or treat a disease. Clinical trials often compare a new treatment to a standard one.

Combination chemotherapy: The use of more than one drug to treat cancer.

Complete blood count (CBC): The number of red blood cells, white blood cells, and platelets in a sample of blood. Also called blood count.

Computed tomography: An imaging procedure in which multiple x-rays are taken of a part of the body to produce cross-sectional images of internal organs. Except for injection of a dye (needed in some but not all cases), this is a painless procedure that can be performed in an outpatient clinical setting. It is often referred to as a "CT" or "CAT" scan.

Contracture: A capsule or shell of dense scar-like tissue that may form around a breast implant. (See also capsule formation).

Core needle biopsy: Removal of tissue or fluid from a lump or cyst with a large needle and syringe.

Cyst: A fluid-filled sac that is usually benign (non-cancerous). The fluid can be removed for analysis. (See needle aspiration).

Cytology: The study or examination of cells by a cyto-pathologist using a microscope to determine whether they are cancerous or benign (non-cancerous).

Cytotoxic: Toxic to cells; cell-killing.

D

Deoxyribonucleic acid (DNA): A long molecule that contains genetic information in all living cells.

Detection: Finding disease. Early detection means that the disease is found at an early stage, before it has grown large or spread to other sites. (Many forms of cancer can develop to an advanced stage without causing symptoms. Because of this, ovarian and pancreatic cancers, for example, are very difficult to detect). Women participate in early detection by performing monthly breast self-examination and getting medical attention for lumps or abnormalities in the breast, by having clinical breast exams by a health professional, and by having mammograms once they reach 40 years of age. Mammography is the principal way to detect breast cancer early. A mammogram can show a developing breast tumor before it can be felt by the woman herself or even by a highly skilled health care professional.

Diagnosis: Identifying a disease by its signs, symptoms, imaging procedures, and/or laboratory findings. In general, the earlier a diagnosis of cancer is made, the better the chance for long-term survival.

Diagnostic mammography: An x-ray examination of the breast in a woman who either has a breast complaint (for example, a breast lump found during self-exam or nipple discharge) or has had an abnormality found during screening mammography. Diagnostic mammography is more involved and time-consuming than screening mammography and is used to determine exact size and location of breast abnormalities and to image the surrounding tissue and lymph nodes. Typically, several additional views of the breast are imaged and interpreted during diagnostic mammography. See also mammography.

Digital mammography: Digital mammography uses essentially the same mammography system as conventional mammography, but the system is equipped with a digital receptor and a computer instead of a film cassette. Digital mammography provides many benefits over standard mammography equipment, including faster image acquisition, shorter exam time, easier image storage, physician manipulation of breast images for more accurate detection of breast cancer, and transmittal of images over phone lines or a network for remote consultation with other physicians. Currently, only one digital mammography system is FDA approved and is not yet widely available. Many physicians predict increased use of digital mammography in the future.

Dimpling: A pucker or indentation of the skin; on the breast, it may be a sign of cancer.

Diuretic: Drugs that help the body get rid of excess water and salt.

Discharge (nipple): Any fluid coming from the nipple. It may be clear, milky, blood, tan, gray, or green. White, yellow, or green nipple discharges are usually benign. Bloody, watery, red, pink, brown, or black nipple discharge may indicate malignancy. Nipple discharge should be evaluated by a physician.

Dissection: Surgery to divide, separate, or remove tissues. (See also axillary dissection).

DNA: Abbreviation for deoxyribonucleic acid. DNA holds genetic information on cell growth, division, and function.

Docetaxel: Brand name, Taxotere. Drug used to treat metastatic breast cancer in patients who have not responded well to standard chemotherapy. Docetaxel inhibits the division of breast cancer cells by acting on the cells' internal skeleton.

Double tier scarring: Term used to describe a standard scar that appears on the breast after TRAM flap breast reconstruction. See also TRAM flap.

Doubling time: The time it takes for a cell to divide and double itself. The doubling time of breast cancer cells depends on many things, such as the type of tumor, the resistance of the individual's body, and the location in which it tries to grow. A single cell needs 30 doublings to reach noticeable size (1 cm)—a billion cells. Cancers vary in doubling time from 8 to 600 days, averaging 100 to 120 days. Thus, a cancer may be present for many years before it can be felt. (See also cell).

Duct: A hollow passage for gland secretions. In the breast, a passage through which milk passes from the lobule (which makes the milk) to the nipple.

Duct ectasia: Widening of the ducts of the breast, often related to breast inflammation called periductal mastitis. Duct ectasia is a benign (not cancerous) condition. Symptoms of this condition are nipple discharge, swelling, retraction of the nipple, or a lump that can be felt.

Ductal carcinoma in situ (DCIS): Cancer cells that start in the milk passages (ducts) and have not penetrated the duct walls into the surrounding tissue. This is a highly curable form of breast cancer that is treated with surgery or surgery plus radiation therapy. Also called intraductal carcinoma.

Ductogram: See galactogram.

Dysplasia: A group of cells that are abnormal in size, shape, appearance, and organization, but which are not yet cancerous.

E

Electrical Impedance Imaging (EIS or T-Scan): A diagnostic test that measures how electricity travels though tissue. Electrical impedance imaging has been approved for use in conjunction with mammography to investigate breast abnormalities. Also called Transscan or T-scan.

Ellence: Generic name, epirubicin. Drug used to treat early stage breast cancer after breast surgery in patients whose cancer has spread to the axillary lymph nodes.

Endocrine glands: Glands that release hormones into the bloodstream. The ovaries are one type of endocrine gland.

Endocrine therapy: Manipulation of hormones for therapeutic purposes. (See also hormone therapy).

Engorgement (breast): Breast swelling that can occur when the breasts produce more milk than the amount that is being expelled by breast-feeding, pumping, or manual (hand) expression. A common problem for breast-feeding mothers, especially during the first two to five days after childbirth.

Epidemiology: The study of factors that have an impact on health and diseases by collecting and analyzing statistical data. In the field of cancer, epidemiologists are studying how many people have cancer; who gets specific types of cancer; and what factors (such as environment, job hazards, family patterns, and personal habits, such as smoking and diet) play a part in the development of cancer.

Epirubicin: Brand name, Ellence. Drug used to treat early stage breast cancer after breast surgery in patients whose cancer has spread to the axillary lymph nodes.

Estrogen: A female sex hormone produced primarily by the ovaries, and in smaller amounts, by the adrenal cortex. In women, levels of estrogen fluctuate on nature's carefully orchestrated schedule, regulating the development of secondary sex characteristics, including breasts; regulating the monthly cycle of menstruation; and preparing the body for fertilization and reproduction. In breast cancer, estrogen may promote the growth of cancer cells. (See estrogen receptor assay, estrogen replacement therapy).

Estrogen receptor assay: Growth of normal breast cells and some breast cancers are stimulated by estrogen. Estrogen receptors are molecules that function as cells' "welcome mat" for estrogen circulating in the blood. Breast cancer cells without these receptors (called estrogen receptor negative or ER-negative) and may be less likely to respond to hormonal therapy. ER-positive cancers are more likely to respond to hormonal therapy. The estrogen receptor assay is a laboratory test done on a piece of the cancer in order to see whether estrogen receptors are present. (See also progesterone receptor assay).

Estrogen replacement therapy (ERT): The use of exogenous estrogen (estrogen not produced by the body; estrogen from other sources) after the body has ceased to produce it because of natural or induced menopause. This type of hormone therapy is often prescribed to alleviate symptoms of menopause and has been shown to provide protective effects against heart disease and osteoporosis in post-menopausal women. Since estrogen nourishes some types of breast cancer, scientists are working on the question of whether estrogen replacement therapy increases breast cancer risk. There appears to be an emerging consensus that estrogen replacement therapy does not significantly increase the risk for breast cancer. This appears to be true for women who are on estrogen less than five years or who take less than 0.625 mg per day. (See also estrogen, menopause, osteoporosis). Some new drugs called selective estrogen receptor modulators (SERMs) are being studied. They seem to have many of the beneficial effects of estrogen replacement without increasing breast cancer risk. Recent studies suggest that some SERMs may actually reduce breast cancer risk. (See also estrogen, menopause, osteoporosis).

Etiology: The cause of a disease. In cancer, there are probably many etiologies, although research is showing that both genetics and lifestyle are major factors in many cancers.

Evista: Generic name, raloxifene. Drug used to prevent and treat osteoporosis. Evista is also being studied to determine whether it can safely and effectively prevent breast cancer in women at high risk for the disease since it is chemically similar to the drug tamoxifen.

Excisional biopsy: The removal of the entire suspected breast lump and a surrounding margin of normal tissue.

Exemestane: Brand name, Aromasin. Drug used to treat metastatic breast cancer in post-menopausal women. Works by binding to the body's aromastase enzyme, an enzyme responsible for producing the hormone, estrogen.

F

False negative: Term used to describe an incorrect test result of a medical procedure or test that falsely shows the lack of a finding. For example, a mammogram may not show any breast abnormality, yet breast cancer is present. The mammogram result is a false negative. A false negative result can occur for a variety of reasons, including operator error or limitations of the test.

False positive: Term used to describe a test result that wrongly or inaccurately shows the presence of a disease or other conditions when none exist.

Fascia: A sheet or thin band of fibrous tissue that covers muscles and various organs of the body.

Fat necrosis: The death of fat cells, usually following injury. Fat necrosis is a benign (non-cancerous) condition, but it can cause a breast lump, pulling of the skin, or skin changes that can be confused with breast cancer.

Fenretinide: A non-toxic drug related to Vitamin A. Researchers are investigating whether fenretinide may reduce the risk of breast cancer recurrence in pre-menopausal women.

Fibroadenoma: A type of benign (non-cancerous) breast tumor composed of fibrous tissue and glandular tissue. On clinical examination or breast self-examination, it usually feels like a firm, round, smooth lump. These usually occur in young women.

Fibrocystic change: A term that describes certain benign (non-cancerous) changes in the breast; also called fibrocystic disease. Symptoms of this condition include cysts (accumulated packets of fluid), fibrosis (formation of scar-like connective tissue), lumpiness, areas of thickening, tenderness, or breast pain. Because these signs sometimes mimic breast cancer, diagnostic mammography or microscopic examination of breast tissue may be needed to show that there is no cancer.

Fibrosis: Formation of fibrous (scar-like) tissue. This can occur anywhere in the body.

Filgrastim: A drug used to treat neutropenic patients (those with a decreased white blood cell count). Brand name, Neupogen.

Fine needle aspiration: Removal of tissue or fluid from a lump or a cyst with a thin needle and a syringe. (See also needle aspiration).

Flap: Term used to describe the transfer of skin and soft tissue from one part of the body to help reconstruct another part. In most instances the flap is attached to the body by its blood supply. The place where the flap is taken from (harvested) is called the donor site. The place on the body where the flap is transferred to is called the recipient site (for example, the breast).

Flap donor sites: The location on the body that a flap of tissue is taken from for breast reconstruction. For example, in a TRAM flap procedure, tissue is taken from the abdomen and transferred to the breast (the recipient site) to reconstruct the breast after a mastectomy.

Follow-up care: After primary breast cancer treatment, patients are usually monitored with mammograms and other tests.

Flow cytometry: A test of tumor tissue to see how fast the tumor cells are reproducing and whether the tumor cells contain a normal or abnormal amount of DNA. This test is used to help predict how aggressive a cancer is likely to be. (See also ploidy, DNA, S-phase fraction).

"Free" flap: Term used to describe a breast reconstructive procedure that is completely detached from its donor site and transferred to the recipient site by reattaching the blood vessels of the flap (tissue) to vessels of the recipient site. For example, in a TRAM flap procedure, tissue is taken from the abdomen (donor site) and transferred to the breast (recipient site) to reconstruct the breast after a mastectomy. Also called microvascular flap.

Frozen section: Microscopic examination of a specimen of tissue that has been quick-frozen. This method gives a quick diagnosis, sometimes while the surgeon is waiting to complete a procedure. The diagnosis is confirmed in a few days by a more detailed study called a permanent section.

G

Galactocele: A clogged milk duct; a cyst filled with milk. It may occur in the breast during breast-feeding.

Galactogram: A special type of contrast enhanced mammography used for imaging the breast ducts. Galactography can aid in diagnosing the cause of an abnormal nipple discharge and is valuable in diagnosing intraductal papillomas (wart-like, non-cancerous tumors with branchings or stalks that have grown inside the breast duct).

Gene: A segment of DNA that contains information on hereditary characteristics such as hair color, eye color, and height as well as susceptibility to certain diseases. Women who have BRCA1 or BRCA2 gene mutations (defects) have an inherited (genetic) tendency to develop breast cancer.

Genetic: Related to or caused by the genes. (See also gene).

Glands: Organs that produce and release substances used locally or elsewhere in the body.

Goserelin acetate: Brand name, Zoladex. Drug used to treat metastatic breast and prostate cancers. Goserelin acetate works by blocking estrogen from breast cancer cells (and blocking testosterone in men), thereby starving these cells.

Grade: The grade of a breast cancer reflects how abnormal it looks under the microscope. There are several grading systems for breast cancer, but all divide cancers into those with the greatest abnormality (grade 3 or poorly differentiated), the least abnormality (grade 1 or well differentiated) and intermediate features (grade 2 or moderately differentiated). Grading is done by the pathologist who examines the biopsy specimen. It is important because higher grade cancers tend to grow and spread more quickly and have a worse prognosis. A cancer's histologic grade is based on features of individual cells as well as how the cells are arranged together.

Granular cell: Usually found in the mouth or skin but may rarely be detected in the breast. Most granular cell tumors of the breast are identified as movable, firm lumps, measuring between 0.5 inch and 1.0 inch in diameter.

Graphic stress telethermometry (GST): A method of measuring surface heat from a distance. Some have used this method, plus computer analysis of heat patterns in the breast, to measure breast cancer risk. This is not a reliable method and is not in standard practice.

Gross Description/"The Gross": Characteristics of a breast biopsy sample that the pathologist measured and felt when examining the tissue with the naked eye (without a microscope).

Gynecologist: A physician who specializes in women's health.

Gynecologist oncologist: A physician who specializes in cancers of a woman's reproductive organs.

H

Halsted radical mastectomy: See mastectomy.

Hematologist: A physician who specializes in diagnosis and treatment of conditions which occur in the blood and blood-forming tissues, including bone marrow.

Hematoma: A collection of blood outside a blood vessel caused by a leak or injury. Hematomas that occur in the breast after injury or after surgery may feel like a lump. As with other breast lumps, it's important to have this checked to be sure that it is indeed a hematoma and not a symptom of a more serious problem.

HER2 or HER-2/neu: Human epidermal growth factor receptor 2; a protein receptor found on the surface of cells. HER2 is a key component in regulating cell growth. When the HER2 gene is altered, extra HER2 receptors may be produced. This over-expression of HER2 causes increased cell growth and reproduction, often resulting in more aggressive tumor cells. Advanced breast cancer patients who over-express the HER2 gene may be treated with the drug, Herceptin. See also Herceptin.

Herceptin (generic name, trastuzumab): A drug used to treat advanced breast cancer patients whose tumors over-express the HER2 growth factor. See also HER2 or HER-2/neu.

Hereditary cancer syndrome: Conditions associated with cancers that occur in multiple family members, because of an inherited, mutated gene.

High risk: Having a higher risk of developing cancer, compared with the general population. See also risk factor.

Histologic grading: The pathologist will assign a histologic grade to a breast tumor upon examination that helps to identify the type of tumor present and the patient's prognosis. See also grade.

Histologic section: The preparation of tissue specimens for microscopic examination.

Histology: The anatomical study of the microscopic structure of tissues, including cellular structure and function. See also histologic sectioning and histologic grading.

Hormone: A chemical substance released into the body by the endocrine glands, such as the thyroid, adrenal, or ovaries. The substance travels through the bloodstream and controls the actions of certain cells of organs in the body. For example, prolactin, which is produced in the pituitary gland, begins and sustains the production of milk in the breast after childbirth.

Hormone receptor assay: A test to see whether a breast tumor is likely to be affected by hormones or if it can be treated with hormones. See also estrogen receptor assay, progesterone receptor assay.

Hormone replacement therapy (HRT): The use of estrogen and/or progesterone from an outside source after the body has stopped producing these hormones. See estrogen replacement therapy for a more detailed explanation.

Hormone therapy: Treatment with hormonal drugs that interfere with hormone production or hormone action, or surgical removal of hormone-producing glands to kill cancer cells or show their growth. The most common hormonal therapy for breast cancer is the drug tamoxifen. Other hormonal therapies include megestrol, aminoglutethimide, androgens and surgical removal of the ovaries (oophorectomy). See also tamoxifen.

Hyperplasia: An abnormal increase in the number of cells in a specific area, such as the lining of the breast ducts or the lobules. By itself, hyperplasia is not cancerous, but when the proliferation (rapid growth) is marked and/or the cells are atypical (unlike normal cells), the risk of cancer developing is greater.

Hypertrophic scarring: This type of scar can occur after a surgical incision. A very severe form of a scar, it actually grows into normal uninvolved skin and does not resolve over a period of time. Also called keloid.

Hysterectomy: An operation to remove the uterus, through an incision in the abdomen or the vagina. Removal of the ovaries (oophorectomy) may be done at the same time. (See also oophorectomy).

I

Imaging: Any method used to produce a picture of internal body structures. Some imaging methods used to detect cancer are x-rays (a breast x-ray is called a mammogram), magnetic resonance (MR) imaging, scintigraphy, computed tomography (CT) imaging, and ultrasonography. (See also mammogram, bone scan, computed tomography, magnetic resonance imaging, ultrasonography).

Immune system: The complex system by which the body resists infection by microbes (such as bacteria or viruses) and rejects

142

transplanted tissues or organs. The immune system may also help the body fight some cancers. (See also antibody, antigen, lymph nodes).

Immunocytochemistry or immunohistochemistry: A laboratory test that uses antibodies to detect specific chemical antigens in cells or tissue samples viewed under a microscope. This procedure can be used to help detect and classify cancer cells. It is also one of the methods used for estrogen receptor assays and progesterone receptor assays. (See also monoclonal antibodies).

Immunology: Study of how the body resists infection and certain other diseases. Knowledge gained in this field is important to cancer treatments based on the principles of immunology. (See also immunotherapy).

Immunosuppression: A state in which the ability of the body's immune system to respond is decreased. This condition may be present at birth, may be caused by certain infections (such as human immunodeficiency virus or HIV), or by certain cancer therapies, such as cytotoxic (cancer-cell killing) drugs, radiation, and bone marrow transplant action.

Immunotherapy: Treatments that promote or support the body's immune system response to a disease, such as cancer.

Incisional biopsy: The removal of part of a lump for microscopic (pathologic) examination. (See also biopsy).

Infiltrating ductal carcinoma (IDC): Cancer beginning in the milk ducts of the breast and penetrating the wall of the duct, invading the fatty tissue of the breast and possibly other regions of the body. IDC is the most common type of breast cancer, accounting for 80% of breast cancer diagnoses. Also called invasive ductal carcinoma.

Infiltrating lobular carcinoma (ILC): Cancer beginning in the milk glands (lobules) of the breast, but often spreading to other regions of the body. ILC accounts for 10% to 15% of breast cancers. Also called invasive lobular carcinoma.

Inflammatory carcinoma: The appearance of inflamed breasts (red and warm) with dimples and/or ridges caused by the infiltration of tumor cells into the lymphatics.

Infraclavicular nodes: Lymph nodes located beneath the clavicle (collar bone).

Inframammary fold: The lower breast fold that attaches the lowest portion of the breast to the rib cage.

Infusion: The slow intravenous (through the vein) delivery of drugs or fluids.

Injection: The use of a syringe and needle to push fluids or drugs into the body. Also called shot.

In situ: Literally meaning, "in place." The term, in situ, applies to cancer that is within the original tissue and has not yet broken through any boundaries between tissues. (See also ductal carcinoma in situ, lobular carcinoma in situ).

Interferon: A protein produced by cells, interferon helps regulate the body's immune system, boosting activity when a threat, such as a virus, is detected. Scientists have learned that interferon helps fight against cancer, so it is used for immunotherapy of some types of cancer.

Internal mammary nodes: Lymph nodes beneath the breast bone on each side. Some breast cancers may spread to these nodes.

Intraductal papilloma: Small, finger-like, polyp-like, noncancerous growths in the breast ducts that may cause a bloody nipple discharge. These are most often found in women 45 to 50 years of age. When many papillomas exist, breast cancer risk is slightly increased.

Intravenous (IV): A method of supplying fluids and medications, using a needle inserted in a vein.

Invasive cancer: Cancer that has spread beyond the area it originally developed in, to involve adjacent tissues. For example, invasive breast cancers develop in milk glands (lobules) or milk passages (ducts) and spread to the adjacent fatty breast tissue. Some invasive cancers spread to distant areas of the body (metastasize), but others do not. Also called infiltrating cancer. (See also invasive ductal carcinoma, invasive lobular carcinoma).

Invasive ductal carcinoma: A cancer that originates in the milk passages (ducts) of the breast and then breaks through the duct wall, where it invades the fatty tissue of the breast. When it reaches this point, it has the potential to spread (metastasize) elsewhere in the breast, as well as to other parts of the body through the bloodstream and lymphatic system. Invasive ductal carcinoma is the most common type of breast cancer, accounting for about 80% of breast malignancies. Also known as infiltrating ductal carcinoma.

Invasive lobular carcinoma: A cancer that arises in the milk-producing glands (lobules) of the breast and then breaks through the lobule walls to involve the adjacent fatty tissue. From this site, it may then spread elsewhere in the breast. About 15% of invasive breast cancers are invasive lobular carcinomas. It is often difficult to detect by physical examination or even by mammography. Also called infiltrating lobular carcinoma.

Inverted nipple: A condition in which the nipple is tucked into the areola (pigmented region surrounding the areola).

Involved margins: Term used to describe breast cancer that extends beyond the surgical margin of removal. This condition indicates that additional cancer is still present in the breast.

K

Keloid: This type of scar can occur after a surgical incision. A very severe form of a scar, it actually grows into normal uninvolved skin and does not resolve over a period of time. Also called hypertrophic scarring.

L

Lactation: Production of milk in the breast.

Large core biopsy: The surgical removal of a substantial sample of breast tissue for pathological examination. Large core biopsy usually removes more breast tissue than vacuum-assisted biopsy but less than open surgical biopsy. The Advanced Breast Biopsy Instrumentation (ABBI) system made by U.S. Surgical is a large core biopsy procedure.

Latissimus dorsi flap procedure: A method of breast reconstruction that uses the long flat muscle of the back, by rotating it to the chest area.

Lesion: A wound, injury, or other damage to a body part. Breast tumors are often referred to as lesions.

LCIS: See lobular carcinoma in situ.

Leukine: Generic name, sargramostim. A drug used to treat neutropenic patients (those with a decreased white blood cell count).

Limited breast surgery: Also called lumpectomy, segmental excision, or tylectomy. It removes the breast cancer and a small amount of tissue around the cancer, but preserves most of the breast. It is almost always combined with axillary lymph node removal and is followed by radiation therapy. (See also lumpectomy).

Linear accelerator: A machine used in radiotherapy to treat cancer. A linear accelerator generates gamma rays and electron beams which are focused on the cancerous tissue.

Lobe: A group of lobules (glands) in the breast. The breast contains 15 to 24 lobes.

Lobular carcinoma in situ (LCIS): A very early type of breast cancer that develops within the milk-producing glands (lobules) of the breast and does not penetrate through the wall of the lobules. Though technically a Stage 0 breast cancer (the earliest stage, many physicians do not classify LCIS as a cancer. However, LCIS places a woman at increased risk of developing an invasive breast cancer later in life, which can occur in either breast.

Lobule: Gland in the breast responsible for producing milk.

Localized breast cancer: A cancer that starts in the breast and is confined to the breast.

Lump: Any kind of mass in the breast or elsewhere in the body. Also called nodule.

Lumpectomy: Surgery to remove the breast tumor and a small margin of surrounding normal tissue. (See also breast conservation therapy, two-step procedure).

Lymph: Clear fluid that passes within the lymphatic system and contains cells known as lymphocytes. These cells are important in fighting infections and may also have a role in fighting cancer.

Lymph nodes: Small bean-shaped structures of immune system tissue such as lymphocytes, located along lymphatic vessels. They remove waste and fluids from lymph and help fight infections. Also called lymph glands. (See also lymph, lymphatic system).

Lymph node removal: Surgery to remove some or all of the lymph nodes. See axillary node dissection, sentinel node biopsy.

Lymphatic system: The tissues and organs (including bone marrow, spleen, thymus, and lymph nodes) that produce and store lymphocytes (cells that fight infection) and the channels that carry the lymph fluid. The entire lymphatic system is an important part of the body's immune system. Invasive cancers sometimes penetrate the lymphatic vessels and metastasize (spread) to lymph nodes.

Lymphedema: A side effect that occurs in some patients after breast cancer treatment; more likely if some or all of the axillary lymph nodes are removed. Swelling in the arm caused by excess fluid that collects after lymph nodes and vessels are removed by surgery or treated by radiation. This condition is usually persistent.

Lymphoma: A cancer of lymphocytes (a type of white blood cell) that usually develops in the lymph nodes. About 5% of cancers are lymphomas. The two main types of lymphomas are Hodgkin's disease and non-Hodgkin's lymphomas. Lymphoma can occur as a result of some types of cancer therapies.

M

Macrocalcifications: Coarse calcium deposits in the breasts, larger than microcalcifications. Macrocalcifications are associated with benign (non-cancerous) conditions and do not typically require a breast biopsy. Macrocalcifications are found in approximately 50% of women over the age of 50.

Magnetic resonance (MR or MRI) imaging: A method of obtaining cross-sectional images of the inside of the body. Instead of using x-rays, MRI uses a powerful magnet and transmits radio waves through the body; the images appear on a computer screen as well as on film. Like x-rays, the procedure is physically painless, but some people

147

find it psychologically uncomfortable to spend 30 minutes or more in the small core of the MRI machine. Also called nuclear magnetic resonance (NMR).

Magnification mammography views: Uses a small magnification table to bring the breast closer to the x-ray source and further away from the film plate. This allows the acquisition of "zoomed in" images (2 times magnification) of the region of interest. Magnification views provide a clearer assessment of the borders and the tissue structures of a suspicious breast area or a mass and are often used to evaluate microcalcifications.

Malignancy: Term used to describe a mass of cancer cells. Malignant tumors may invade surrounding tissues or spread (metastasize) to distant areas of the body. See cancer.

Mammastatin: A protein that is being studied in connection with breast cancer prediction and treatment. Mammastatin is thought to be a naturally occurring protein produced by breast cancer cells. The protein was first identified in 1986 and has been determined in preliminary research to be lacking in the majority of breast cancer patients and healthy women who have a family history of breast cancer.

Mammoplasty: Plastic surgery to reconstruct the breast or to change the shape, size, or position of the breast. Reduction mammoplasty reduces the size of the breast(s). Augmentation mammoplasty enlarges the size of the breast(s), usually with implants.

Mammogram, mammography: An x-ray of the breast; used to screen for or investigate breast abnormalities and breast cancer, particularly those which are too small to be felt by physical examination. Mammograms are made using a special x-ray machine designed specifically for this purpose. Screening mammography is used for early detection of breast cancer in women without any breast symptoms. Diagnostic mammography is used to help characterize suspicious breast masses or determine the cause of other breast symptoms.

Mass: Any group of cells clustered together more densely than the surrounding breast tissue. Masses can be palpable (able to be felt) or nonpalpable (unable to be felt). Masses can be benign or malignant.

Mastalgia: Cyclic or non-cyclic pain in the breast or in the axilla (underarm) region of the body. Approximately 15% of women with breast pain require treatment. Breast pain is not usually (but can be) associated with breast cancer.

Mastectomy: Surgery to remove all or part of the breast and sometimes other tissue. Extended radical mastectomy removes the breast, skin, nipple, areola, chest muscles (pectoral major and minor), and all axillary and internal mammary lymph nodes on the same side. Halsted radical mastectomy removes the breast, skin, nipple, areola, both pectoral muscles, and all axillary lymph nodes on the same side. Modified radical mastectomy removes the breast, skin, nipple, areola, and most of the axillary lymph nodes on the same side, leaving the chest muscles intact. Partial mastectomy removes less than the whole breast, taking only part of the breast in which the cancer occurs and a margin of healthy breast tissue surrounding the tumor. Subcutaneous mastectomy is surgery to remove internal breast tissue. The nipple and skin are left intact. Prophylactic mastectomy is a mastectomy done before any evidence of cancer can be found, for the purpose of preventing cancer. This procedure is sometimes performed on women at very high risk of breast cancer. Quadrantectomy is a partial mastectomy in which the quarter of the breast that contains a tumor is removed. Segmental mastectomy is a partial mastectomy. Simple mastectomy or total mastectomy removes only the breast and areola.

Mastitis: Inflammation or infection of the breast.

Mastopexy: Surgery to lift sagging breasts. The procedure is not permanent.

Medical oncologist: See oncologist.

Medullary carcinoma: A special type of infiltrating ductal carcinoma with especially sharp boundaries between tumor tissue and normal tissue. About 5% of breast cancers are medullary carcinomas. The outlook (prognosis) for this kind of cancer is considered to be better than average.

Menarche: A woman's first menstrual period. Early menarche (before age 12) is a risk factor for breast cancer, possibly because the earlier a woman's periods begin, the longer her exposure to estrogen.

Menopause: The time in a woman's life when monthly cycles of menstruation cease forever and the level of hormones produced by the ovaries decreases. Menopause usually occurs in the late 40s or early 50s, but it can also be caused by surgical removal of both ovaries (oophorectomy), or by some chemotherapies that destroy ovarian function. (See also estrogen replacement therapy).

Metachronous: At different times. (See also bilateral).

Metastasis: The spread of cancer cells to distant areas of the body by way of the lymph system or bloodstream. 25% of metastatic breast cancer spreads first to the bone.

Metastatic breast cancer: Cancer cells that have spread past the breast and the axillary lymph nodes to distant regions of the body (such as the bone, liver, lung, or brain).

Microcalcifications: See calcifications.

Micrometastases: The spread of cancer cells in groups so small that they can only be seen under a microscope.

Microvascular flap: A surgical technique that reattaches the small vessels of the flap to the small recipient site vessels. See also "free" flap.

Modified radical mastectomy: See mastectomy.

Monoclonal antibodies: Antibodies manufactured in the laboratory and designed to seek out as targets specific substances recognized by the immune system (antigens). Monoclonal antibodies which have been attached to chemotherapy drugs or radioactive substances are being studied for their potential to seek out antigens unique to cancer cells and deliver these treatments directly to the cancer, thus killing the cancer cell and not harming healthy tissue. Monoclonal antibodies are often used in immunocytochemistry to help detect and classify cancer cells. Other studies are being done to see if radioactive atoms attached to monoclonal antibodies can be used in imaging tests to detect and locate small groups of cancer cells. (See also antibody, antigen, immunocytochemistry).

Monomorphic: Of the same shape. Monomorphic often describes microcalcifications that are uniform in shape and density (and usually non-cancerous).

Mucinous carcinoma: A tumor that is sticky because of a large amount of mucin released by its cells. Mucin is a carbohydrate that is the main component of mucus.

150

Multicentric breast cancer: Breast cancer occurring in multiple areas of a breast.

Multiform: Having an irregular shape or various shapes. Term often used to describe microcalcifications, which can indicate ductal carcinoma in situ (DCIS), an early stage breast cancer.

Myocutaneous flap: A flap of tissue that consists of skin, fatty and muscle tissue from a place in the body (such as the abdomen) that is used to reconstruct the breast.

N

Necrosis: Term used to describe the death of cellular tissue. Necrosis within a cancerous tumor may indicate that the tumor is growing so rapidly that blood vessels are not able to multiply fast enough to nourish some of the cancer cells. Necrosis usually indicates that the tumor is very aggressive and can spread quickly. Fat necrosis is a benign (non-cancerous) breast condition that may occur when fatty breast tissue swells or becomes tender spontaneously or as the result of an injury to the breast.

Needle aspiration: A type of needle biopsy. Removal of fluid from a cyst or cells from a tumor. In this procedure, a needle and syringe (like those used to give injections) is used to pierce the skin, reach the cyst or tumor, and with suction, draw up (aspirate) specimens for biopsy analysis. If the needle is thin, the procedure is called a fine needle aspiration or FNA. (See also needle biopsy).

Needle biopsy: Removal of fluid, cells, or tissue with a needle for examination under a microscope. There are two types: fine needle aspiration (also called FNA or needle aspiration) and core biopsy. FNA uses a thin needle and syringe (like those used to give injections) to pierce the skin and draw up (aspirate) fluid or small tissue fragments from a tumor. A core needle biopsy uses a thicker needle to remove a cylindrical sample of tissue from a tumor.

Needle localization: Also called wire localization. A procedure used to guide a surgical breast biopsy when the breast lump is difficult to locate or in areas that look suspicious on the x-ray (mammogram) but do not have a distinct lump. Mammogram or ultrasound images are used to guide the needle to the suspicious area of the breast. The radiologist typically replaces the needle with a wire and sends the patient to the surgeon with only a wire in place. The surgeon then uses the path of the wire as a guide to locate the abnormal area to be removed. Needle localization is usually used when there is no palpable (able to be felt) lump (i.e., a finding found only or most convincingly on an imaging study such as a mammogram or ultrasound.

Neoadjuvant therapy: Treatment such as chemotherapy or hormonal therapy that is given to a patient prior to surgery. Neoadjuvant therapy may help shrink breast tumors so that they may be removed with a less complicated surgical procedure.

Neoplasm: An abnormal growth (tumor) that starts from a single altered cell, a neoplasm may be benign (non-cancerous) or malignant (cancerous). Cancer is a malignant neoplasm.

Neupogen: Generic name, filgrastim. A drug used to treat neutropenic patients (those with a decreased white blood cell count).

Neutropenia: An abnormal decrease in white blood cells most often resulting from a viral infection or exposure to certain drugs or chemicals. Neutropenia may be a side effect of chemotherapy.

Nipple: The tip of the breast; the pigmented projection in the middle of the areola. The nipple contains the opening of milk ducts from the breast. The nipple consists mainly of skin and ductal breast tissue.

Nipple confusion: A fairly common condition in which the baby becomes "confused" between the mother's nipple and an artificial nipple of a bottle. Babies with nipple confusion will not latch on to the mother's nipple and become fussy when a mother tries to breast-feed.

Nipple discharge: Any fluid coming from the nipple. It may be clear, milky, bloody, tan, gray, or green.

Nodal status: Indicates whether a breast cancer has spread (node-positive) or has not spread (node-negative) to lymph nodes in the armpit (axillary nodes). The number and site of positive axillary nodes can help predict the risk of cancer recurrence.

Node: See lymph node.

Nodule: A small, solid lump that can be located by touch. Also called mass or nodule.

Nolvadex: Trade name for tamoxifen; an antiestrogen drug commonly used in breast cancer therapy. (See also antiestrogen, tamoxifen, hormonal therapy).

Noncancerous: Benign; no cancer is present; not malignant.

Noninvasive breast cancer: Cancer cells that are confined to the breast ducts and do not invade surrounding fatty and connective tissues of the breast. Ductal carcinoma in situ (DCIS) is the most common form of noninvasive breast cancer (90%). Lobular carcinoma in situ (LCIS) is less common and considered a marker for increased breast cancer risk.

Nonpalpable: A breast abnormality that is present but unable to detect by touch. Mammography helps detect many nonpalpable breast cancers in an early stage.

Normal hormonal changes: Changes in breast and other tissues that are caused by fluctuations in levels of female hormones during the menstrual cycle.

Nuclear magnetic resonance (NMR): See magnetic resonance imaging.

Nuclear medicine scan: A method for localizing diseases of internal organs such as the brain, liver, or bone, in which small amounts of a radioactive substance (isotope) are injected into the bloodstream. The isotope is concentrated in certain organs. A scintillation (nuclear medicine) camera is used to produce an image of the organ and detect areas of disease.

Nucleus: The center of a cell where the DNA is housed and replicated. Studying the size and shape of a cell's nucleus under the microscope can help pathologists distinguish breast cancer cells from benign (non-cancerous) breast cells.

Nulliparous: A woman who has never given birth to a child.

Nurse practitioner: A registered nurse (RN) who has completed additional courses and specialized training. Nurse practitioners can work with or without the supervision of a physician. They take on additional duties in diagnosis and treatment of patients, and in many states they may write prescriptions. (See also oncology nurse specialist).

153

Nursing: Giving a baby milk from the breast. Also called breast-feeding or suckling.

O

Oncogene: A type of gene. When these genes are abnormally "turned on" (activated), they cause excessive growth and other characteristics of malignancy.

Oncologist: A physician who is specially trained in the diagnosis and treatment of cancer. Medical oncologists specialize in the use of chemotherapy and other drugs to treat cancer. Radiation oncologists specialize in the use of x-rays and other radiation to kill tumors. Surgical oncologists specialize in performing operations to remove cancer.

Oncology: The branch of medicine that deals with cancer and tumors.

Oncology nurse specialist: A registered nurse who has taken additional courses and specialized training in the care of cancer patients. Oncology nurse specialists may prepare and administer treatments, monitor patients, prescribe and provide aftercare, and teach and counsel patients and their families. Some oncology nurse specialists are also certified nurse practitioners. (See also case manager, nurse practitioner).

Oncology social worker: A person with a master's degree in social work who has specialized in working with cancer patients. The oncology social worker provides counseling and assistance to people with cancer and their families, especially in dealing with the non-medical crises that can result from cancer, such as financial problems, housing when treatments must be taken at a facility far away from home, and child care.

One-step procedure: Surgery during which the procedure to diagnose the presence of breast cancer (see biopsy) is followed immediately by treatment (such as mastectomy—removal of the breast). The patient is given general anesthesia and does not know until she wakes up if the diagnosis was cancer or if a mastectomy was performed. Once the only option in breast cancer treatment, the one-step procedure is now rarely used. (See also two-step procedure).

Oophorectomy: Surgery to remove the ovaries, the primary source of estrogen. It may be performed to remove a lump, tumor, or

154

abscess, or to treat endometriosis. Oophorectomy is also a preventive measure to reduce the risk of breast cancer by stopping the production of estrogen.

Osteoporosis: Breakdown of bone, resulting in diminished bone mass and reduced bone strength. Osteoporosis can cause pain, deformity (especially of the spine), and fractures (broken bones). This condition is common among post-menopausal women. (See also estrogen replacement therapy).

Ovarian cancer: A cancer of the ovary. The ovary is one of the pair of female sexual reproductive organs (gonads) found on each side of the lower abdomen, beside the uterus. Ovarian cancer occurs in approximately one in 55 women.

Ovary: Reproductive organ in the female pelvis. Normally a woman has two ovaries. They contain the eggs (ova) that, when joined with sperm, result in pregnancy. Ovaries are also the primary source of estrogen.

P

p53 gene: A gene that normally helps to suppress tumors, researchers have found that, when mutated, the p53 gene increases a woman's risk of developing breast cancer.

Paclitaxel (brand name, Taxol): See Taxol.

Paget's disease of the nipple: A rare form of breast cancer that begins in the milk passages (ducts) and spreads to the skin of the nipple and areola. This affected skin may appear crusted, scaly, red, or oozing. The prognosis is generally better if these nipple changes are the only sign of breast disease and no lump can be felt.

Palliative treatment: Therapy that relieves symptoms, such as pain, but is not expected to cure the disease. Its main purpose is to improve the patient's quality of life.

Palpable: Able to be felt.

Palpation: The examination of the breasts by manually feeling for breast lumps. A palpable mass in the breast is one that can be felt.

Parenchyma: The functional tissue of an organ. In the breast, it is the glandular tissue, as opposed to fatty or stromal (connective) tissues.

Partial mastectomy: See mastectomy.

Pathologist: A physician who specializes in examining, diagnosing, and classifying diseases by conducting laboratory tests (such as examining tissues and cells under a microscope). The pathologist determines whether a lump is benign or cancerous.

Pectoral muscles: Muscles attached to the front of the chest wall and upper arms. The larger one is called pectoralis major, and a smaller one is called pectoralis minor. Because these muscles are next to the breast, breast cancer may occasionally spread to the pectoral muscles.

Pectoralis muscle: The main chest wall muscle that is underneath the breast tissue.

Per os (PO): By mouth, orally. Denotes a medication or treatment given orally.

Pathology: Branch of science that deals with all aspects of disease, specifically the microscopic examination of body tissue to look for **evidence of disease.**

Peripheral neuropathy: A condition of the nervous system that usually begins in the hands and/or the feet with symptoms of numbness, tingling, and/or weakness. Can be caused by certain anticancer drugs.

Permanent section: Preparation of tissue for microscopic examination. The tissue is soaked in formaldehyde, processed in various chemicals, surrounded by a block of wax, sliced very thin, attached to a microscope slide and stained. This usually takes 1-2 days. It provides a clear view of the specimen so that the presence or absence of cancer can be determined. (See also frozen section).

Phyllodes tumors: Breast tumors that may be found in the glandular and stroma (connective) tissues of the breast. Phyllodes tumors are usually benign but on very rare occasions, they may be cancerous. Also spelled phylloides.

Physician: A licensed medical doctor or doctor of osteopathy (DO) who typically participates in additional training (a residency) after medical school to specialize in a more limited field of practice.

Placebo: An inert or inactive substance that is not distinguishable from the active substance. Placebos are often used in clinical trials to compare the effects of a given treatment with no treatment.

Plastic surgeon: A physician with advanced training in cosmetic surgery. Plastic surgeons may surgically reconstruct a woman's breast after mastectomy (breast removal).

Platelets: Type of blood cells that help stop bleeding.

Pleomorphic: Having many or various shapes. These terms often describe microcalcifications which can indicate ductal carcinoma in situ (DCIS), an early stage breast cancer.

Ploidy: A measure of the amount of DNA contained in a cell. Ploidy is a characteristic (marker) that helps predict how aggressive a cancer is likely to be. Cancers with the same amount of DNA as normal cells are called diploid and those with either more or less than that amount are aneuploid. About two-thirds of breast cancers are aneuploid.

Polymorphic: Having an irregular shape or various shapes. This term often describes microcalcifications which can indicate ductal carcinoma in situ (DCIS), an early stage breast cancer.

Postmenopause: Term used to describe the time in a woman's life after menopause.

Precancerous: Abnormal changes in cells that indicate a higher than normal risk of developing into cancer. (See also premalignant).

Predisposition: Susceptibility to a disease that can be triggered under certain conditions. For example, some women have a family history of breast cancer and are therefore predisposed (but not necessarily destined) to develop breast cancer.

Premalignant: Abnormal changes in cells that may, but do not always, become cancer. Also called precancerous.

Premenopause: Term used to describe the time in a woman's life before menopause.

Prevalence: A measure of the proportion of persons in the population with a particular disease at a specified time.

Primary cancer: The site where cancer begins. Primary cancer is usually named after the organ in which it originates (for example, cancer that originates in the breast is always breast cancer even if it metastasizes to other organs, such as bones or lungs).

Progesterone: A female sex hormone released by the ovaries during every menstrual cycle to prepare the uterus for pregnancy and stimulate milk production (lactation) in the breast.

Progesterone receptor assay: A laboratory test done on a piece of the breast cancer to determine whether the cancer depends on progesterone for growth. Progesterone receptors are tested along with estrogen receptors for more complete information on the hormone sensitivity of a cancer, and how best to treat it. (See also estrogen receptor assay).

Prognosis: A prediction of the course of disease; the outlook for the cure of the patient. For example, a woman with breast cancer that was detected early and received prompt treatment generally has a good prognosis.

Prolactin: A hormone released from the pituitary gland that prompts milk production (lactation).

Prophylactic mastectomy: See mastectomy.

Prosthesis: An artificial form, such as a breast prosthesis, that can be worn under the clothing after a mastectomy. (Plural: prostheses).

Protocol: A formalized outline or plan such as a description of what type of treatments a patient will receive and exactly when each should be given.

Ptosis: The natural droop of the breast over the inframammary fold.

R

Radical (Halsted or standard) mastectomy: See mastectomy.

Radiodense: Effective in blocking x-rays. Breast tissue in younger women is usually more "radiodense" than the fattier tissue in older women. Some contrast agents used in various x-ray procedures are also radiodense. Also called radiopaque.

Radioisotope: Also called isotope. A type of atom that is unstable and prone to break up (decay). Decay releases small fragments of atoms and energy. Exposure to certain radioisotopes can cause cancer. Use of radioisotopes under controlled conditions can be used to treat cancer (see radiotherapy). In certain nuclear medicine imaging procedures, radioisotopes are injected. They travel through the body and collect in areas where the disease is active, showing up as highlighted areas on the images (see nuclear medicine scan). In breast cancer, radioisotopes are used to check for metastasis to the bones.

Radiologic technologist: A health professional (not a physician) trained to properly position patients for x-rays or other radiology studies such as CT or mammography, perform the imaging study, and to develop and check the images for quality. Since mammograms (breast x-rays) are done on a machine that is used only for mammograms, the technologist must have special training in mammography. The films taken by the technologist are sent to a radiologist to be read.

Radiologist: A physician who has taken additional training in interpretation of x-rays and other types of diagnostic imaging studies (for example, mammography, ultrasound, magnetic resonance imaging, computerized axial tomography, etc.) (See imaging).

Radiopaque: Effective in blocking x-rays. Breast tissue in younger women is usually more "radiopaque" than the fattier tissue in older women. Some contrast agents used in various x-ray procedures are also radiopaque. Also called radiodense.

Radiotherapy/radiation therapy: Treatment with radiation to destroy cancer cells. External sources of radiation used include linear accelerators, cobalt, and betatrons. This type of treatment may be used to reduce the size of a cancer before surgery, or to destroy any remaining cancer cells after surgery. Also called radiation therapy and irradiation. See also internal radiation or bracytherapy.

Raloxifene: Brand name, Evista. Drug used to prevent and treat osteoporosis. Raloxifene is also being studied to determine whether it can safely and effectively prevent breast cancer in women at high risk for the disease since it is chemically similar to the drug tamoxifen.

Reconstruction: See breast reconstruction.

Reconstructive mammoplasty: See mammoplasty, latissimus dorsi flap procedure, and transverse rectus abdominus muscle flap procedure.

Reconstructive surgery: See breast reconstruction.

Rectus abdominus flap procedure: See transverse rectus abdominus muscle flap procedure.

Recurrence: Cancer that returns after treatment. Local recurrence occurs at the same site as the original cancer. Regional recurrence occurs in the lymph nodes near the site of origin. Distant recurrence occurs in organs or tissues further from the original site than the regional lymph nodes (such as the lungs, liver, bone marrow, or brain). The term, metastasis, is used to describe a disease has recurred at another site in the body.

Red blood cells: Cells that supply oxygen to tissues throughout the body.

Reduction mammoplasty: See mammoplasty.

Regimen: A strict, regulated plan (such as diet, exercise, or other activity) designed to reach certain goals. In cancer treatment, a plan to treat cancer.

Regional involvement: The spread of breast cancer from its original site to nearby areas such as the axillary lymph nodes, but not to distant sites such as other organs.

Rehabilitation: Activities to adjust, heal, and return to a full, productive life after injury or illness. This may involve physical restoration (such as the use of prostheses, exercises, and physical therapy), counseling, and emotional support.

Relapse: Reappearance of cancer after a disease-free period. See recurrence.

Remission: Complete or partial disappearance of the signs and symptoms of cancer in response to treatment; the period during which a disease is under control. A remission may not be a cure.

Residual breast tissue: The remaining glandular breast tissue still in the treated breast following breast-conserving surgery (lumpectomy).

Revision surgery: A second surgery that may be needed to modify the results of the original breast reconstructive or cosmetic surgery.

Risk factor: Anything that increases a person's chance of getting a disease, such as cancer. Known risk factors for breast cancer include: family history of the disease especially in one's mother or sister; beginning menstrual periods at a young age (early menarche) and ending periods at an older age (later menopause); and obesity.

S

Saline breast implant: Breast implant filled with a salt-water solution. (See also breast implant).

Saline: A sterile solution of salt (sodium chloride) and water. Medical saline is typically the same salinity ("saltiness") as blood.

Sarcoma: A malignant tumor growing from connective tissues, such as cartilage, fat, muscle, or bone. Several types of sarcoma (such as angiosarcoma, liposarcoma, and malignant phylloides tumor) can rarely develop in the breast, and they differ in their prognosis.

Sargramostim: Brand name, Leukine. A drug used to treat neutropenic patients (those with a decreased white blood cell count).

Scan: A study using either x-rays, radioactive isotopes or magnetic resonance to produce images of internal organs and structure of the body. (See also bone scan, brain scan, computed tomography (CT) scan, magnetic resonance imaging (MRI), nuclear medicine scan).

Scar: The healing response by the body to any form of injury.

Scarff-Bloom-Richardson grading system: The most common type of cancer grade system currently used by physicians. Breast tumors are assigned a grade of 1, 2, or 3 based on observed features of the tumor.

Scintillation camera: Device used in nuclear medicine scans to detect radioactivity and produce images that help diagnose cancer and other diseases.

Screening: The search for disease, such as cancer, in people without symptoms. Screening may refer to coordinated programs in large populations. The principal screening measure for breast cancer is mammography.

Screening mammography: See mammography, screening.

Secondary tumor: A tumor that forms as a result of spread (metastasis) of cancer from its site of origin.

Segmental mastectomy: See mastectomy.

Segmental resection: See mastectomy.

Sentinel node biopsy: A new procedure that involves removing only the sentinel node(s), the first lymph node in the lymphatic chaining, to determine whether the breast cancer has spread to the lymph nodes. Research has shown the sentinel node biopsy can significantly reduce lymphedema (arm swelling), the most common side effect of axillary node dissection.

Seroma: Clear fluid trapped in the wound. A seroma usually forms after breast cancer surgery, filling the surgical cavity after the operation and naturally remolding the breast's shape. Gradually, the seroma is absorbed by the body.

Shot: The use of a syringe and needle to push fluids or drugs into the body. Also called injection.

Side effects: Results of a drug or other form of therapy in addition to the intended effect, such as hair loss caused by chemotherapy and fatigue caused by radiation therapy.

Silicone gel: Synthetic material used in breast implants because of its flexibility, strength, and texture, which is similar to the texture of the natural breast. Silicone gel breast implants are available for women who have had breast cancer surgery, but only if they participate in a clinical trial. (See also breast implant).

Simple mastectomy: See mastectomy.

Skin dimpling: Indentations of the breast skin, possible indication of breast cancer. See also dimpling.

Sonography: See ultrasound.

S-phase fraction (SPF): The percentage of cells that are replicating their DNA. DNA replication usually indicates that a cell is getting ready to split into two new cells. A low SPF is a sign that a tumor is slow-growing; a high SPF shows that the cells are dividing rapidly and the tumor is growing quickly.

Spiculated: On a mammogram, dense regions with radiating lines that suggest breast masses or distortions. The term is used to describe highly suspicious masses that may indicate cancer. However, some post-operative scars may be quite spiculated and resemble cancer.

Spot compression mammography: An x-ray view of the breast that apply the compression to a small area of tissue using a small compression plate or cone. By applying compression to only a specific area of the breast, the effective pressure is increased on that spot. This results in better tissue separation and allows better visualization of the small breast area in question. Also called compression mammogram, spot view, cone views, or focal compression views.

Staging: The process of determining and describing the extent of cancer. Staging of breast cancer is based on the size of the tumor, whether regional axillary lymph nodes are involved, and whether distant spread (metastasis) has occurred. Knowing the stage at diagnosis is essential in selecting the best treatment and predicting a patient's outlook for survival.

Standard therapy, standard treatment: See therapy.

Statistically significant: Term used to describe a scientifically proven relationship that is the result of an objective analysis in a large group of patients.

Stereotactic needle biopsy: A method of needle biopsy that is useful in some cases in which calcifications or a mass can be seen on mammogram but cannot be located by touch. Computerized equipment maps the location of the mass and this is used as a guide for the placement of the needle. (See also needle aspiration, needle biopsy).

Stomatitis: Inflammation or ulcers of the mouth area. This condition can result as a side effect of some chemotherapy regimens.

Subcutaneous mastectomy: See mastectomy.

Suckling: Giving a baby milk from the breast. Also called breast-feeding or nursing.

Supraclavicular nodes: Lymph nodes that are above the collarbone (clavicle).

Surgeon: A physician with a medical doctorate (MD) degree and advanced training in surgical techniques. Some surgeons specialize in a specific area of the body (for example, the breast). Surgeons perform breast biopsy, lumpectomy, and mastectomy on breast cancer patients.

Survival rate: The percentage of people who live a certain period of time. For example, the 5-year survival rate for women with localized breast cancer (including all women living five years after diagnosis, whether the patient was in remission, disease-free, or under treatment) was 78% in the 1940s, but in the l990s, it is over 97%.

Suspicious: A breast abnormality that may indicate breast cancer. On a mammogram, these abnormalities may be lesions such as spiculated masses or pleomorphic microcalcifications.

Synchronous: At the same time. (See also bilateral).

Systemic disease: In breast cancer, this term means that the tumor that originated in the breast has spread to distant sites, such as the liver, brain, bones, or lungs.

Systemic therapy: Treatment that reaches and affects cells throughout the body as opposed to targeting one specific area; for example, chemotherapy.

Tamoxifen (brand name, Nolvadex): This drug blocks the effects of estrogen on many organs, such as the breast. Blocking estrogen is desirable in some cases of breast cancer because estrogen promotes their growth. Recent research suggests that tamoxifen may lower the risk of developing breast cancer in women with certain risk factors.

T

Taxol (generic name, paclitaxel): A drug sometimes used to treat breast cancer that has spread into and/or beyond the axillary (underarm) lymph nodes.

Taxotere: Generic name, docetaxel. Drug used to treat metastatic breast cancer in patients who have not responded well to standard chemotherapy. Taxotere inhibits the division of breast cancer cells by acting on the cells' internal skeletons.

Therapy: Any measure taken to treat a disease. Unproven therapy is any therapy that has not been scientifically tested and approved. Use of an unproven therapy instead of standard therapy is called alternative therapy. Taking vitamin supplements or herbs to help treat breast cancer is an example of an alternative therapy. Some alternative therapies have dangerous or even life-threatening side effects. For others, the main danger is that a patient may lose the opportunity to benefit from standard therapy. Complementary therapy, on the other hand, refers to therapies used in addition to standard therapy. Some complementary therapies may help relieve certain symptoms of cancer, relieve side effects of standard cancer therapy, or improve a patient's sense of well-being. Patients should discuss alternative or complementary therapies with their physician before beginning them.

Thermography: A method in which heat from the breast is measured and mapped. Also called a thermogram or thermal imaging, this method is not yet reliable in detecting breast cancer.

Thrush: A yeast infection that develops in the baby's mouth and is characterized by white patches on the baby's tongue, gums, and cheeks inside the mouth. Thrush most commonly results from antibiotics taken by the mother or baby.

Tissue: A collection of cells, united to perform a particular function.

Tissue expander: A device used to stretch the remaining breast skin after a mastectomy. A tissue expander is similar to a balloon, and the surgeon will fill the expander with salt-water solution periodically (usually once a week). The expansion process typically takes three to four months. After the skin is sufficiently stretched, the surgeon will replace the expander with a permanent breast implant. Also called breast expander.

TMN classification: The most commonly used method of breast cancer staging classification currently used by physicians. The TMN system assigns a stage to a breast cancer (0-IV) based on tumor size (T), palpable nodes (N), and/or extent of spread (mestatasis, M).

Total mastectomy: See mastectomy.

TRAM flap: See transverse rectus abdominus muscle flap procedure.

Transillumination: See diaphanography.

Transscan: See electrical impedance imaging.

Transverse rectus abdominus muscle flap procedure: A method of breast reconstruction in which tissue from the lower abdominal wall which receives its blood supply from the rectus abdominus muscle is used. The tissue from this area is moved up to the chest to create a breast mound and usually does not require an implant. Moving muscle and tissue from the lower abdomen to the chest results in flattening of the lower abdomen (a "tummy tuck"). Also called a TRAM flap or rectus abdominus flap procedure.

Trastuzumab (brand name, Herceptin): See Herceptin.

T-Scan: See electrical impedance imaging.

Tumor: A growth (lump or mass) which has formed due to excessive accumulation of abnormal cells. "Tumor" is not a precise medical term. Tumors can be benign (not cancerous) or malignant (cancerous).

Two-step procedure: A method in which the breast biopsy for diagnosis and breast surgery for treatment (such as lumpectomy or mastectomy, if the diagnosis is breast cancer) are performed as two separate procedures, after an interval of days or weeks. This method is strongly preferred by women and their health care teams because it allows time to consider all options. (See also one-step procedure).

Tylectomy: See lumpectomy.

U

Ultrasonography (ultrasound): An imaging method that uses high-frequency waves to image the breast or other parts of the body. High-frequency sound waves are transmitted from a transducer through the area of the body being studied. The sound wave echoes are picked up and displayed on a computer monitor or television screen. Ultrasound is a painless method that is sometimes useful in distinguishing fluid-filled cysts from solid tumors. Ultrasound involves no exposure to radiation.

Unifocal: Term used to describe cancer that is present in only one spot in the breast.

Unilateral: Affecting one side of the body. For example, unilateral breast cancer occurs in only onVaccine: Inactivated, killed, or weakened disease-causing organisms (for example, mumps or measles virus) that are injected into the body for the purpose of developing resistance to the disease. The body's immune system responds to the vaccine by forming antibodies and activating certain immune system cells that are specifically targeted to those particular organisms. The result is that the body is then resistant (immune) to the disease for a specific period of time; in some cases, the immunity lasts forever. Development of a cancer vaccine is a subject of intense research. (See immune system and antibody).

V

Vaginitis: Any inflammation (swelling) of the vagina. Atrophic vaginitis is an inflammation of the vagina in which the vaginal tissue becomes thin and dry. This condition may occur after menopause due to a lack of estrogen. (See also menopause.) An estrogen cream may be prescribed to relieve this problem. Vaginitis can also be a side effect of chemotherapy.

Valley view: Also called "cleavage view," it is a mammogram view of the most medial portions of the breasts. This is the portion of breast tissue "in the valley" between the two breasts.

W

White blood cells: Several types of blood cells that help defend the body against infections from bacteria, viruses, parasites, and foreign tissue such as abnormal or tumor cells. Certain cancer treatments (particularly chemotherapy) can reduce the number of these cells and make a patient more vulnerable to infections. Some types of white blood cells may also help the body fight certain cancers. (See also neutropenia).

Wire localization: Also called needle localization. A procedure used to guide a surgical breast biopsy when the breast lump is difficult to locate or in areas that look suspicious on the x-ray (mammogram) but do not have a distinct lump. Mammogram or ultrasound images are used to guide the needle to the suspicious area of the breast. The radiologist typically replaces the needle with a wire and sends the patient to the surgeon with only a wire in place. The surgeon then uses the path of the wire as a guide to locate the abnormal area to be removed. Needle localization is usually used when there is no palpable (able to be felt) lump (i.e., a finding found only or most convincingly on an imaging study such as a mammogram or ultrasound.

X

X-rays: One form of radiation that can, at low energy levels, produce an image of the body or organ on film or computer monitor using a special detector. At high energy levels, x-rays can be used to destroy cancer cells.

Xeroradiography (xeromammography): An outdated form of mammography that records the image of the breast on paper rather than on film. This method is rarely used now.

Z

Zoladex: Generic name, goserelin acetate. Drug used to treat metastatic breast and prostate cancers. Zoladex works by blocking estrogen from breast cancer cells (and blocking testosterone in men), thereby starving these cells.

About the Author

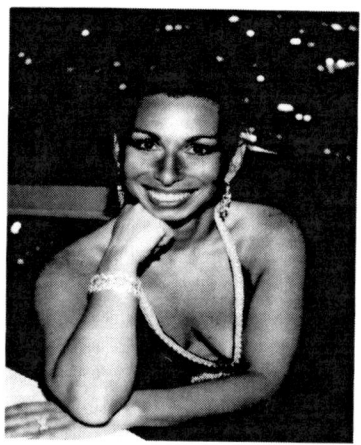

Stacey Chillemi has an Associate Degree in business, a BA in marketing and a minor in advertising. She has worked for NBC, Dateline, Channel 4 News, and other large companies. And has always had a strong background in Business and Marketing. She has also written speeches/proposals for other people speaking in front of congress. MY ACCOMPLISHMENTS: She is a H.O.P.E. Mentor, for the Epilepsy Foundation. Spoken at different events for schools, organizations, political events, and in front of Congress in Washington and anywhere her help is needed to educate people about epilepsy. She was on four talk shows. The interviews focused on the importance of understanding what epilepsy is, how to help someone having a seizure and giving people with epilepsy encouragement and hope for the future. Stacey has been on radio stations discussing epilepsy and appeared in many newspapers all over New Jersey such as, The Leader, Belleville Post and the Star Ledger. In addition, on June 26, 2002, she was presented an award by the Epilepsy Foundation of New Jersey for Outstanding Volunteer Award. She has received awards and certificates in recognition for outstanding efforts in trying to improve society and been an active participant in organizations and activities. She has been a role model to many individuals. She has written many published articles and has appeared three times on News 12 on the talk show New Jersey Women and has had articles written about her efforts to help people with epilepsy. She has contributed time to helping people with epilepsy and making society more aware of the disorder. Websites:
http://www.lulu.com/staceychillemi
http://www.authorsden.com/staceydchillemi

169

BOOKS PUBLISHED BY STACEY CHILLEMI:

1. The Complete Herbal Guide: A Natural Approach to Healing the Body
2. Epilepsy You're Not Alone
3. Eternal Love: Romantic Poetry Straight from the Heart
4. My Mommy Has Epilepsy (Children's Book)
5. My Daddy Has Epilepsy (Children's Book)
6. Keep the Faith: To Live and Be Heard from the Heavens Above (poetry book)
7. Live, Learn, and Be Happy with Epilepsy
8. Epilepsy and Pregnancy: What Every Woman Should Know
   Co-authored by Dr. Blanca Vasques
9. Faith, Courage, Wisdom, Strength and Hope
10. How to Be Wealthy Selling Informational Products on the Internet
11. How to Become Wealthy in Real Estate
12. How to Become Wealthy Selling Ebooks
13. Life's Missing Instruction Manual: Beyond Words

STACEY CHILLEMI STORIES AND POETRY HAVE BEEN PUBLISHED IN:

- **Chicken Soup for the Recovering Soul**
- **Chicken Soup for the Shoppers Soul**
- **Whispers of Inspiration**

ACCOMPLISHMENTS:

- H.O.P.E. Mentor, for the Epilepsy Foundation
- Speaker at different events for schools, organizations, political events
- Spoke in front of Congress in Washington for employment discrimination for people with epilepsy
- Appeared on four talk shows to discuss epilepsy focusing on the importance of understanding epilepsy, how to help someone having a seizure and giving people with epilepsy encouragement and hope for the future.
- Appeared on radio stations discussing epilepsy
- Appeared on the Michael Dressor Show – Health Radio
- Appeared in newspapers all over New Jersey such as, The Leader, Belleville Post and the Star Ledger.

- June 26, 2002, I was honored an award by the Epilepsy Foundation of New Jersey for Outstanding Volunteer Award.
- Received awards in my achievements and certificates in recognition for outstanding efforts in trying to improve society.
- Active participant in organizations and activities.
- Published over 400 articles.
- Author has a dynamic personality and strong public speaking skills.

References

Marisa C. Weiss, M.D. is the Founder, President and guiding force behind breastcancer.org, the world's most trafficked online resource for medically-reviewed breast health and breast cancer information, reaching over 8 million visitors per year. A breast cancer oncologist with twenty years of active practice in the Philadelphia region, Dr. Weiss is regarded as a visionary advocate for her innovative and steadfast approach to informing, empowering, and treating patients with breast cancer.

Dr. Weiss has been honored and recognized as:

- Founder and President of breastcancer.org

- Appointed member of the National Cancer Institute Director's Consumer Liaison Group since April 2000

- Founder and past President (1990-2000) of Living Beyond Breast Cancer® (LBBC), a national nonprofit education and support organization

- Author of the acclaimed book *Living Beyond Breast Cancer* (Random House, 1997 and 1998)

- Selected Doctor of the Year 2005 by Philadelphia Magazine, with a cover feature article on the doctor-patient relationship

- Honored several times by the American Cancer Society and as 2003 Professor of Survivorship Award from the Susan G. Komen Foundation

- Professional advisory board member of Mommy's Light Lives On, nonprofit organization

- Professional advisory board member of the Philadelphia Wellness Community

- Keynote speaker on the international women's health conference circuit, including Speaking of Women's Health, WebMD and breastcancer.org

- Member of the American Society of Clinical Oncology and the American Society of Therapeutic Radiation Oncology

- Past board member of the National Breast Cancer Coalition

Dr. Weiss's media appearances and affiliations include:

- Regular contributor for ABC News, has authored several articles for the network's website and is frequently called upon as a medical expert

- Guest appearances on CNN House Call during Breast Cancer Awareness Month for three consecutive years (2003-2006)

- Co-producing and/or guest appearing on the NBC Today Show's Special Breast Cancer Series for seven consecutive years (1998-2004)

- Medical Editor for Lifetime Television film, *Why I Wore Lipstick to My Mastectomy*

- Guest speaker for WebMD's special breast cancer feature (2001-2004)

- Guest appearances on National Public Radio's Fresh Air with Terry Gross and Radio Times with Marty Moss-Cohane, as well as CNNRadio, ABC Radio, CBS Radio, Washington Post Radio, and the radio partner for Cosmopolitan magazine.

- Interviewed and regularly quoted for leading print outlets including The New York Times, USA Today, The Wall Street Journal, The Washington Post, The Philadelphia Inquirer, and articles for the Associated Press newswire, as well as People, Ladies' Home Journal, Redbook, More, Shape, Self, Allure, and O.

- Serves on the advisory board for Women's Health magazine

Dr. Weiss currently practices at Lankenau Hospital, part of the Main Line Health Hospitals of the Thomas Jefferson University Health System in the Philadelphia-area, where she serves as Director of Breast Radiation Oncology and Director of Breast Health Outreach. After attending the University of Pennsylvania for her undergraduate studies, medical school, residency, and laboratory research fellowship, Dr. Weiss became an assistant professor in Penn's Radiation Oncology Department. In 1992, she established her clinical practice in the Main Line Health System.

Dr. Weiss lives in Wynnewood, Pennsylvania, with her husband, a pediatrician and avid fisherman, their three children, and two dogs.

Robert J. Allen, M.D.

Robert J. Allen, M.D., is the pioneer of the skin sparing DIEP/SIEA/S-GAP flap and the founder of The Center for Microsurgical Breast Reconstruction. As a plastic surgeon, he has an interest in autogenous breast reconstruction and microsurgery. He believes that all women have the chance to keep their stomach muscle and still have natural breasts after breast cancer. Dr. Allen has limited his practice to microsurgical breast reconstruction for the past seven years.

Dr. Allen received a medical degree from the Medical University of South Carolina. He then went on to residency at Louisiana State University in plastics and general surgery. After completion of general and plastic surgery training in Louisiana, he moved to New York City for a one-year fellowship in reconstructive microsurgery at New York University Center. Upon returning to New Orleans, Dr. Allen was appointed to program director of LSU Plastic Surgery Residency. He now holds fellowships with other plastic surgeons who have an interest in learning breast microsurgery.

Jennifer Armstrong, M.D.

Jennifer Armstrong, M.D., is a breast cancer oncologist with Paoli Hematology Oncology Associates in Paoli, Pa. She joined the Professional Advisory Board, she says, because breastcancer.org "is one of the few websites (and organizations) that offers an unbiased perspective on everything patients want and need to know about breast cancer, and then it takes the time to break that down into language that's easy to understand. It's an incredible resource to anyone with breast cancer, or anyone who is trying to be there for someone with breast cancer."

Dr. Armstrong received her B.A. from the University of Pennsylvania and her M.D. from Penn's School of Medicine. She did her internship and residency in Internal Medicine at the Hospital of the University of Pennsylvania. A Fellow at Weill Medical College of Cornell University and at Memorial Sloan-Kettering Cancer Center (MSKCC), both in New York, she received MSKCC's Brian Piccolo Memorial Fellowship, awarded annually to a Fellow focusing in breast cancer research.

Dr. Armstrong has a special interest in physicians' communication skills. She is Founder and Co-Facilitator of a Ballint Group for Medical Oncology Fellows that discusses the stresses of clinical oncology and also focuses on communication skills training. She previously served on a Steering Committee at MSKCC charged with developing curricula to improve physicians' communication skills.

Katrina Armstrong, M.D., M.S.C.E.

Katrina Armstrong, M.D., M.S.C.E., is Assistant Professor of Medicine, Senior Fellow in the Leonard Davis Institute of Health Economics, and Senior

Scholar in the Center for Clinical Epidemiology and Biostatistics at the University of Pennsylvania School of Medicine. Her research interest is screening and prevention, with particular focus on genetic testing for breast cancer susceptibility, risk communication, and improving decision-making surrounding post-menopausal therapy.

Katrina is an expert on the decision-making process, balancing pros and cons in difficult issues, to help the breastcancer.org audience make sense of the tough choices they face, when no "right answer" seems clear. Her presence on the breastcancer.org website rounds out our expertise and depth on the role of genes and genetic testing.

Dr. Armstrong currently holds a Clinical Research Training Grant from the American Cancer Society and a Measey Foundation Faculty Fellowship, and is a past recipient of a Preventive Oncology Career Development Award from the National Cancer Institute. Her publications include evaluation of the use of hormone replacement in women with BRCA1/2 mutations, cost-effectiveness of raloxifene in post-menopausal women, access to medications over the Internet, breast cancer risk assessment, and the relationship between ethnicity and use of BRCA1/2 testing.

José Baselga, M.D.

José Baselga, M.D., is Chief of Medical Oncology Service at the Vall d'Hebron University Hospital, and of Céntro Medico Teknon, both in Barcelona, Spain. He is also Professor of Medicine at the Universidad Autónoma de Barcelona, where he obtained his medical degree, and the Scientific Chairman of the Spanish Breast Cancer Cooperative group SOLTI. After completing residencies in internal medicine in Spain and New York, he did his fellowship in medical oncology at Memorial Sloan-Kettering Cancer Center and then joined its Breast Oncology Service. In 1996 he returned to Spain. Dr. Baselga is an Associate Editor of *Annals of Oncology* and a member of the Editorial Advisor boards for *Clinical Cancer Research* and *Investigational New Drugs*. He has published over 200 abstracts, articles, and book chapters on his research interests, focusing on growth factor receptors and downstream molecules as targets for breast cancer therapy.

"I am enthusiastic about joining the Professional Advisory Board of breastcancer.org," he says. "If we want to defeat this disease, nothing is more important than patient information and society awareness. breastcancer.org is ideally suited to be a great tool for patients and the community."

Norman Berk

Norman Berk is a highly regarded financial planner and investment manager based in Birmingham, Alabama. Trained as an accountant and a lawyer, he devotes his working life to helping people carefully plan their future, preparing for any possibility. He's used to dealing in "what ifs" and "maybes," but when his wife, Phyllis, developed breast cancer, her diagnosis dragged his family into a world of fear and uncertainty none of them had ever before encountered.

Luckily, Phyllis has recovered fully. And Norman, who'd always worked for community charities, decided the time had come to do something about breast cancer in his community. Together with a few others who shared his vision, he created The Breast Cancer Research Foundation to help women and their families obtain the best quality of care in Birmingham. The Foundation has raised more than $650,000 for breast cancer research, all of which has been donated to the Comprehensive Cancer Center at the University of Alabama Birmingham.

Norman joined the breastcancer.org Professional Advisory Board because he wanted to reach beyond his own community and make a significant difference in the lives of women around the world struggling to overcome breast cancer. It was his own visionary thinking and the generosity of The Breast Cancer Research Foundation board that resulted in the Foundation making a gift of the domain name "breastcancer.org" to ibreast.

Kimberly L. Blackwell, M.D.

Kimberly L. Blackwell, M.D., is an Associate in Medicine in the Division of Hematology-Oncology at Duke University Medical Center. As a clinician, she is interested in the hormonal treatment of breast cancer, the treatment of young women with breast cancer, and the effects of exercise and nutrition on the recovery period after chemotherapy. In the laboratory, she studies the effects of hormones on tumor angiogenesis (how tumors develop new blood vessels). She also studies tests for the early detection of breast cancer, and the breast cancer protein made by the HER2/neu cancer gene. She is currently involved in several trials incorporating the use of novel therapies in the treatment of locally advanced breast cancer.

Kim realizes that the hardest times faced by breast cancer survivors are after the "active" therapies are finished. The recovery period from treatment is when laboratory values and radiographs become less important, and patients must face even bigger life and health issues, such as the fear of breast cancer recurrence and long-term effects of chemotherapy. Such issues are not easily addressed during routine doctor's visits. Dr. Blackwell would like to help breastcancer.org develop programs in which dealing with these issues ultimately contributes to the "whole person recovery" of all breast cancer patients.

Rachael Brandt, MS, CGC

Rachael Brandt is a certified genetic counselor and the coordinator of the Cancer Risk Assessment and Genetics Program for Main Line Health Lankenau and Bryn Mawr Hospitals.

Rachael is dedicated to supporting women and families at risk for hereditary breast cancer. To this end, she founded a face-to-face networking group for women with *BRCA1* or *BRCA2* mutations called AWARE (Answers for Women At Risk will Empower).

In addition, Rachael has co-authored several papers and abstracts related to cancer genetics services, breast cancer risk perception, and motivations and concerns among women seeking genetic testing for breast cancer.

After graduating with a BS in Biology from Davidson College, Rachael joined the Institute for Genomic Research as a research and development team member. In addition, she also served within the Genetic Alliance. Upon graduating with an MS in Genetic Counseling from Arcadia University, Rachael began providing cancer genetics consultations under the direction of an internationally known pioneer within the cancer genetics field and has held an adjunct faculty position at Northwestern University.

"It is an honor to serve on the Professional Advisory Board of breastcancer.org. I hope to educate women about breast cancer genetics so they have the tools to determine if they or their family members may be at risk. Knowing risk is the first step in breast cancer prevention."

Cecilia M. Brennecke, M.D.

Radiologist Cecilia M. Brennecke, M.D., is Medical Director at Johns Hopkins at Greenspring in Baltimore, Maryland. As a breast imaging specialist, she interprets mammography, performs ultrasound and breast MRI, conducts clinical breast exams, and performs the newest image-guided biopsy procedures.

Dr. Brennecke received her medical degree at the University of Pennsylvania, and completed her residency in radiology at Johns Hopkins Hospital. She has a fellowship in ultrasound.

Aman U. Buzdar, M.D.

Aman U. Buzdar, M.D., is Professor of Medicine at the University of Texas Cancer Center at M.D. Anderson Hospital and Tumor Institute in Houston. He is also Deputy Department Chairman in the Department of Breast Medical Oncology there, and an associate editor of the journal *Clinical Cancer Research*. His research interest lies in improving and defining short- and long-term benefits of chemotherapy, and he is testing several new hormonal therapies in the treatment of breast cancer. Dr. Buzdar was born in Pakistan and maintains many ties there, as indicated by his lifetime achievement award from the Pakistan Society of Clinical Oncology.

"I am thrilled to be able to join my international colleagues in reaching even more women around the world with the best information and guidance on breast cancer," he says of his position on the breastcancer.org Professional Advisory Board.

Robert Carlson, M.D.

Robert Carlson received his medical degree from Stanford University School of Medicine, and did his internship and junior residency in internal medicine at Barnes Hospital in St. Louis. He joined the faculty at Stanford after his fellowship and is Professor of Medicine there, as well as Associate Chief for Clinical Affairs, Division of Oncology. His primary areas of investigation include breast cancer clinical trials and the use of computer-based systems to assist health care providers in the delivery of care. Dr. Carlson is Chair of the Breast Cancer Guidelines Committee and the Breast Cancer Risk Reduction Guidelines Committee for the National Comprehensive Cancer Network.

"Participation in efforts such as breastcancer.org is crucial to effectively educating patients and health care providers about state-of-the-art breast cancer evaluation and treatment," he says. "Together, the educated patient and health care provider make a productive, effective partnership."

Ned Z. Carp, M.D.

Ned Z. Carp, M.D. is Chief of the Division of General Surgery and Director of Surgical Oncology at Lankenau Hospital in Wynnewood, PA. He was a major contributor to the original trials of sentinel lymph node biopsy for women with early stage of breast cancer. Another important research interest of Dr. Carp's is the evaluation of bone marrow to help detect micrometastatic disease.

Dr. Carp is a native Philadelphian who graduated from the University of Pennsylvania and received his Doctor of Medicine from Temple University School of Medicine. He completed his surgical residency at Abington Memorial Hospital and his surgical oncology fellowship at Fox Chase Cancer Center.

He is a Fellow in the American College of Surgeons, a member of the American Society of Clinical Oncology, and the American Society for Gastrointestinal Endoscopy. Dr. Carp is also a member of The American Radium Society, the Society for Surgical Oncology, and a Member of the Eastern Cooperative Oncology Group.

Dr. Carp is on the Breast Committee of the National Surgical Adjuvant Breast Project. He is also on the Breast Committee of the American College of Surgeons Oncology Group.

"I feel that breast cancer.org gives patients access to the cutting edge research regarding breast cancer. Every new advance can be found on this website," Dr. Carp says.

Carol Cherry, R.N.C, B.S.N., O.C.N.

Carol Cherry, R.N.C, B.S.N., O.C.N., is health educator, Research Project Manager, and Cancer Risk Counselor in the Margaret Dyson Family Risk Assessment Program at the Fox Chase Cancer Center in Pennsylvania. She works closely with women who have a family history of breast and ovarian cancer, to evaluate their risk and explore prevention and genetic testing options. Her prior experience in radiation oncology nursing has provided her with a rich background in the care of breast cancer patients, from diagnosis to terminal care. She says, "Women need accurate, complete information to make informed decisions. I am committed to assisting breastcancer.org in this effort."

Carol was formerly a risk assessment counselor and radiation oncology nurse at the Paoli (Pennsylvania) Cancer Center, beloved by everyone with and for whom she worked. Carol has also worked at the Bryn Mawr and Good Samaritan Hospitals. She was a founding member and President of the Penns Wood Chapter of the Oncology Nursing Society, and has a strong commitment to expanding clinical expertise, for both herself and her colleagues.

Sara Cohen, OTR/L, CLT-LANA

Sara Cohen is an occupational therapist at Memorial Sloan-Kettering Cancer Center in New York City, where she works with patients who have had breast cancer and lymphedema. She is also certified as a lymphedema therapist by the Lymphology Association of North America. She uses a wide range of therapeutic approaches to customize treatment for each person's unique condition. Her main goal is to help her clients assess the impact of lymphedema on their daily lives, and to provide options for managing this frustrating and perplexing condition. She co-authored the article "Lymphedema: Strategies for Management" published in a supplement to the journal *Cancer* in August 2001.

"What I find most satisfying and enjoyable about working with my clients with lymphedema," she says, "is listening to each woman's unique story and helping her make choices about her treatment, because there is not one simple answer for how to manage lymphedema."

Emily Conant, M.D.

Emily Conant, M.D., is Chief of Breast Imaging at the University of Pennsylvania Medical Center in Philadelphia. She is a pioneer in the development of digital mammography, and a leader in research on the use and benefits of early mammography screening and on the role of MRI and PET scanning. She is also the recipient of grants from the National Institutes of Health to compare standard surgical biopsy with digital mammography and stereotactic core breast biopsy (biopsy guided by an imaging study). *Philadelphia Magazine* named Dr. Conant one of its "Top Docs." She's also been a featured expert in national media including "Good Morning America," CBS News, *USA Today*, *The New York Times*, and *Redbook Magazine*.

"Breast imaging is a rapidly growing field with many new emerging technologies that have improved our ability to detect and diagnose breast cancer at its earliest and most curable stage," Dr. Conant says. "breastcancer.org provides an invaluable opportunity to inform women about these imaging studies so they can ask the questions necessary to obtain the highest quality testing available."

Kenneth H. Cowan, M.D., Ph.D.

Dr. Kenneth Cowan is Director of the Eppley Cancer Center and the Eppley Institute for Research in Cancer and Allied Diseases at the University of Nebraska Medical Center in Omaha. Prior to this position, he spent his entire career at the National Cancer Institute in Bethesda, where, beginning in 1988, he served as chief of the Medical Breast Cancer Section, Medicine Branch. In his NCI position, he led a team of 12 laboratory researchers and a clinical staff of six performing trials in patients with breast cancer. His research focuses on the mechanisms of drug resistance, the biology of breast cancer, and gene therapy.

In 2002, Dr. Cowan was one of seven scientists appointed by the President as a representative to the National Cancer Advisory Board (NCAB). The NCAB advises the Secretary of the Department of Health and Human Services and the Director of the NCI on the activities of the Institute.

Mary Daly, M.D., Ph.D.

Mary Daly, M.D., Ph.D., is Director of the Family Risk Assessment Program at the Fox Chase Cancer Center in Philadelphia. She has devoted her career to the understanding of and education for breast cancer and ovarian cancer risk issues, for individuals and their families. She is a devoted and beloved physician and a distinguished clinical scientist, producing important studies on prevention and options for patients at genetic risk, reaching beyond the local scene to many different institutions to get big things done.

Mary is quiet and modest, yet passionate and effective in her work. She is on the Board of Scientific Advisors of the National Cancer Institute and the professional advisory board of the Gilda Club. With her interest in reaching out to distant institutions with her research, she is a natural – and valuable – asset to breastcancer.org.

M. Maitland DeLand, M.D.

M. Maitland DeLand, M.D. is a radiation oncologist in Lafayette, La, and is President, Chief Executive Officer and Owner of OncoLogics, Inc., a group of clinical practices throughout Louisiana. She holds hospital staff appointments at several facilities in the state, including the University Medical Center, Our Lady of Lourdes Regional Medical Center and Women and Children's Hospital. She has served on the Tulane Cancer Center Community Advisory Board in New Orleans since 2003 and is a member of the NCI designated cancer consortium in New Orleans.

Dr. DeLand received her B.S. and M.D. from the University of Florida and completed her residency and fellowship in Radiation Oncology at Duke University Medical School. She was awarded an American Cancer Society Clinical Fellowship and is board certified in therapeutic radiology. In 2006 she was recognized with an American College of Radiation Oncology Fellowship and will receive an American College of Radiology Fellowship in 2007.

After watching her patients suffer with radiation dermatitis caused by life-saving radiation therapy for cancer, she recently completed research proving that LED Photomodulation reduces the occurrence and severity of painful dermatitis among her breast cancer patients. In LED Photomodulation, pulsating non-thermal light is directed to the treated area and activates healing cells in the skin, which decreases the enzymes that cause skin breakdown. She presented these results at the American College of Radiation Oncology's (ACRO) 16th annual meeting and the American Society for Laser Medicine & Surgery's (ASLMS) 26th annual meeting. She has also been invited to present these findings at the 2007 International Master Course of Aging Skin (IMCAS) meeting in Paris.

One of Dr. DeLand's major interests is in quality improvement of medical facilities and the establishment of new programs with medical professionals, specialists, and local hospitals. She is proud to serve on the breastcancer.org advisory board because of its continued dedication to helping women and their families with breast cancer find the best medical resources when they need them.

Dianne Dunkelman

Dianne Dunkelman is Founder and President of Speaking of Women's Health, and President and CEO of the National Speaking of Women's Health Foundation, both organizations dedicated to providing women across the United States with cutting-edge medical information, within group discussions and large presentations, "in a warm, enlightening, and entertaining format." As a passionate and committed leader of the women's health movement, Dianne will make certain that every woman who needs breastcancer.org will find breastcancer.org.

Dianne has raised nearly five million dollars for the arts and for health and social service organizations in her adopted hometown of Cincinnati, Ohio. Over the past twenty-five years she has become an expert – and artist – at organizing charity fund- raising events, and her efforts have been recognized throughout the country. In 2004, she was honored with the National

181

Conference for Community and Justice Citation Award. She received the YWCA Career of Achievement Award in 2001 and the Athena Award from the Partnership for Women's Health at Columbia University in 2000. In 1999, Dianne was recognized as one of Cincinnati's Leading Women for her advocacy in women's health, and in 1996 she received the Charles W. Vaughan Award for her work with public television. She was named Cincinnati Enquirer Woman of the Year in 1989, honored with a Post Corbett Award in 1991, and selected by the National Society of Fund Raising Executives for the National Philanthropy Award in 1992. Watch Dianne reach out to women affected by breast cancer in ways we haven't yet dreamed of.

Beth Baughman DuPree, M.D., F.A.C.S.

Dr. Beth DuPree's impressive credentials do not capture the humanitarian spirit with which she treats her patients, friends, and acquaintances. Dr. DuPree, a general surgeon who is focusing her practice on breast cancer care, believes that using a holistic approach to healing a patient is extremely important. It is her position that marrying both holistic therapies with state-of-the-art, leading-edge technology can lead to better outcomes-even in people with life-threatening disease, such as cancer.

Dr. DuPree strongly urges her patients to get alternative healing support, whether it is through clinical psychological therapy, spiritual assistance, grief counseling, exercise programs, reflexology, nutritional counseling, Reiki, Yoga, or massage. In fact, she herself has participated in all and believes that "whatever it takes to help a person find healing and peace is the way to curing them."

This vibrant, witty mother of two sons, whose skin-sparing mastectomies with plastic surgeon Robert Skalicky, D.O., were featured live on the Internet in October 1999, has won numerous awards for her medical work as well as her humanitarian endeavors. The mastectomy Web cast and subsequent television documentary received a Gracie Allen Award in New York City in April 2000. Additionally, Dr. DuPree was given the Clara Barton Humanitarian Award from the American Red Cross in 2002, the Visions of Hope Award in December 2002, the Northampton Township Citizen of the Month in February 2003, and the Women Pioneering the Future Award from the Pennsylvania Commission for Women in March 2003. She is on the advisory committee for Gilda's Club and the Young Survivor's Coalition for Young Breast Cancer Survivors.

Dr. DuPree, who received her medical degree from Hahnemann University in Philadelphia in 1987, is presently writing a book titled *The Healing Consciousness*. She has been the keynote speaker at numerous conferences and seminars, primarily in addressing women's health issues.

A native of York, Pennsylvania, Dr. DuPree lives in Bucks County, Pennsylvania, with her husband Joe and their two sons. Dr. DuPree credits her accomplishments to her family's constant support.

Diana Dyer, M.S., R.D.

Diana Dyer, M.S., R.D., is a Registered Dietitian in Ann Arbor, Michigan, and a two-time breast cancer survivor. Diana is also a survivor of neuroblastoma, a childhood cancer. After a 20-year career working in the specialty area of critical care nutrition, Diana combined her personal experience and professional expertise to focus her efforts on increasing awareness of the benefits of proactively including nutrition as a component of true comprehensive cancer care. Diana also has served as a consultant to the University of Michigan's Integrative Medicine Research Center and is on the Professional Advisory Board for the Wellness Community of Southeast Michigan. She is a board member of the Oncology Nutrition Dietetic Practice Group of The American Dietetic Association, currently serving as Chair of the newly formed Survivorship Subunit. The Michigan Dietetic Association has honored Diana with the Individual Public Relations and Dietitian of the Year Awards. The Oncology Nutrition Dietetic Practice Group of the American Dietetic Association presented Diana with their Distinguished Practice Award in 2005.

"I am honored to be an advisor to breastcancer.org, a leader in providing the reliable information women need to make informed decisions about treatment choices for a breast cancer diagnosis and optimizing health and wellness after breast cancer."

Francene M. Fleegler, M.D.

Francene M. Fleegler, M.D., is Clinical Associate Professor of Medicine at the University of Pennsylvania School of Medicine, and a Preceptor in Oncology at the University's School of Nursing. She is also Director of Hematology/Oncology at Penn Medicine at Radnor. Dr. Fleegler has given twenty invitational lectures and has written an exercise manual with Brooks Johnson called "Coaching Manual" and a book with her physician husband Edward, *The Physician's Guide to Heart Rate Training*.

Dr. Fleegler has wide-ranging professional interests, from diabetes, leukemia, cancer and cancer risk evaluation, and genetic screening, to nutrition, exercise, and cancer prevention. She has become an exercise maven, touting the powerful benefits of exercise to enhance health and well-being. Her next book will present the considerable benefits of exercise for patients with cancer or other serious illness.

Francene is a great role model for what she preaches, and her patients love her. But she's moving to Colorado, so her Philadelphia-area patients – and everyone else – can tap into her wisdom via breastcancer.org.

Silvia C. Formenti, MD

Silvia C. Formenti, M.D., is Professor and Chairman of the Department of Radiation Oncology at the New York University School of Medicine in New

York City. Before joining the NYU faculty in 2000, Dr. Formenti was a tenured Associate Professor of both Radiation Oncology and Medicine at the University of California School of Medicine in Los Angeles.

Dr. Formenti was born in Milan, Italy, and attended medical school at the Universita degli Studi di Milano. She completed residencies in internal medicine, medical oncology radiology and radiation oncology in Milan, before coming to the United States, where she completed an internship in general medicine and residency in radiation oncology before joining the faculty at USC.

Dr. Formenti has been the principal investigator in many important studies, and has recently received multi-year peer-reviewed grants from the American Cancer Society and the Breast Cancer Research Foundation. Her extensive research interests include developing a new model for the treatment of locally advanced breast cancer by assessing the molecular characteristics of tumors before starting treatment; and studying novel treatment regimens including hormonal treatment, chemotherapy, and radiation.

Thomas G. Frazier, M.D.

Thomas G. Frazier, M.D., is Senior Attending Surgeon and Medical Director of the Comprehensive Breast Center at the Bryn Mawr Hospital, and Clinical Professor of Surgery at Thomas Jefferson University in Philadelphia. Much of his education and training was at the University of Pennsylvania's School of Medicine and Hospital, and at M.D. Anderson Hospital in Houston, Texas. Tom's hands-on skills and judgment as a surgeon, and his curiosity and cutting-edge research interests, make him an especially valuable resource for breastcancer.org and the people who come to our site.

He has been a principal investigator for the National Surgical Adjuvant Breast Project (NSABP) since 1976, and a member of both the Commission on Cancer of the American College of Surgeons and the Board of Directors of the NSABP. He is also past president of the Philadelphia Metropolitan Chapter of the American College of Surgeons and president of the Philadelphia Academy of Surgery. Yet along with his busy surgical practice he always finds the time to participate in health education programs in the community. His research interests have included fine needle cytology, ultrasound-guided fine needle aspiration, and sentinel node biopsies for breast cancer, as well as methods for partial breast irradiation (MammoSite brachytherapy).

Patricia A. Ganz, M.D.

Medical oncologist Patricia A. Ganz is a Professor in the schools of Medicine and Public Health at UCLA, and is Director of the Division of Cancer Prevention and Control Research at the Jonsson Comprehensive Cancer Center there.

Her research over the past 20 years has contributed to our understanding of how women adjust to the diagnosis of breast cancer, including its effects on their physical, emotional, social, and sexual well-being. She developed a way to predict which women are likely to develop significant psychological distress in the year following their diagnosis, and has completed several studies examining the quality of life in breast cancer survivors.

"I am delighted to work with an organization that has already done so much for breast cancer survivors and that I know will do more in the future," Patricia says of her role on the breastcancer.org Professional Advisory Board.

With funding from the National Cancer Institute (NCI), Dr. Ganz recently completed a study, "Moving Beyond Cancer," that developed and tested a video that provide successful in helping women more rapidly recover from the effects of breast cancer treatment. This video is available now from the NCI by calling 1-800-4-CANCER. In other studies, funded by the Komen Foundation and the Department of Defense, she examined the impact of breast cancer treatments on reproductive health, cardiovascular function, and osteoporosis in women who were 50 years old or younger when they were treated. Her current research is focused on understanding the biological causes of fatigue, cognitive problems, and sleep disorders in breast cancer survivors.

In July 1999, Dr. Ganz was awarded an American Cancer Society Clinical Research Professorship and honored with the Komen Foundation Professor of Survivorship Award. She currently leads the UCLA-LIVESTRONG Cancer Survivorship Center of Excellence, funded in part by the Lance Armstrong Foundation.

Ronda Gates, M.S., R.Ph.

Ronda Gates, M.S., R.Ph., is an Adult Development specialist and health promotion educator who develops and delivers programs and products to support lifestyle change. Ronda was a hospital pharmacist for seventeen years, then she traded in her white coat for a pair of athletic shoes, created a corporate fitness business, and never looked back. Combining that business experience with graduate education in nutrition, counseling, and life has generated honors from a range of professional organizations including the Association for Worksite Health Promotion and the Oregon Governor's Council for Health, Fitness and Sports.

Ronda describes herself as an "agent for change." She's presented more than five hundred keynote introductions and workshops, and has written or coauthored five books that reached best-seller status, including the most recent, *Beauty, More Than Skin Deep*.

Paul B. Gilman, M.D.

Paul B. Gilman, M.D., has an extensive and distinguished career as an oncologist specializing in breast cancer. He is chief of the division of hematology/oncology at Lankenau Hospital, outside of Philadelphia, and medical director of the hospital's cancer center. He is also an assistant professor of medicine at Jefferson Medical College in Philadelphia, and founded the oncology clinic at St. Joseph's Hospital in Philadelphia in 1985. Additionally, Dr. Gilman is director of the Lankenau Breast Cancer Multidisciplinary Treatment Group. He is known for his warmth with his patients, who leave his office feeling well taken care of and who find numerous opportunities to spread the word of his caring and kindness.

Dr. Gilman received his medical degree from Jefferson Medical College in 1976, completing his residency in internal medicine at New England Deaconess Hospital in Boston, and fellowship training at Thomas Jefferson University Hospital and Temple University Hospital in Philadelphia. He has received a National Cancer Institute grant, and is a principal investigator for several regional oncology group trials.

"Knowledge and information are among the most powerful weapons in the battle against breast cancer," says Dr. Gilman of his participation on the breastcancer.org Professional Advisory Board. "To be able to convey this on a large scale in a highly accessible fashion, beyond traditional confines, is a very exciting opportunity."

Mindy Goldman, M.D.

Mindy Goldman is an OB/GYN physician specializing in the gynecology of Breast Cancer Patients. She is an Associate Clinical Professor of Obstetrics and Gynecology at the University of California, San Francisco's Carol Franc Buck Breast Care Center. She has been on the faculty of UCSF for 8 years as a general Obstetrician/Gynecologist and Associate Director of the OB/GYN Residency Training Program.

Dr. Goldman completed her medical training at the University of Vermont and OB/GYN Residency at UCSF. She has been recognized for her excellence in teaching both locally and nationally and has received several teaching awards from medical students and residents. Dr. Goldman was recently awarded an Outstanding Contributions Award in Education by the UCSF Department of OB/GYN.

Dr. Goldman is also the co-founder and co-chair of the Board of Directors for the Uilani Fund. This nonprofit organization provides financial support for alternative and complementary treatments for women with breast cancer to help them improve the quality of their lives.

Dr. Goldman's life changed when her best friend got breast cancer. She never expected that as a gynecologist, she would develop a practice that focuses on women's health issues for breast cancer patients, but her experience with her friend's cancer was life- altering. "As more and more women live with breast cancer, quality of life issues become so vital," she says. "I am excited to be part of an organization that is dedicated to providing education for women with breast cancer. It is such an amazing resource and can truly affect the lives of so many."

William J. Gradishar, M,D.

Dr. William J. Gradishar is Associate Professor of Medicine in the Division of Hematology and Medical Oncology, Department of Medicine, at the Feinberg School Medicine at Northwestern University in Chicago, Illinois. His research focuses on the development of the latest therapies for breast cancer treatment. He has published numerous articles in the area of breast cancer therapy, with a focus on new endocrine therapy and chemotherapy.

After receiving his medical degree from the University of Illinois Abraham School of Medicine in Chicago, he completed a residency and chief residency in internal medicine at Michael Reese Hospital and Medical Center in Chicago. He then went on to a fellowship in medical oncology at the University of Chicago.

Dr. Gradishar is a member of the Robert H. Lurie Comprehensive Cancer Center of Northwestern University. He also serves as Director of Breast Medical Oncology, Associate Director of the Lynn Sage Comprehensive Breast Program, and Program Director of Northwestern University's Hematology/Oncology Fellowship Training Program.

In addition, he is a Fellow of the American College of Physicians, a member of the American Association for Cancer Research and the American Federation for Clinical Research. He chairs the Oncology Training Program Committee of the American Society of Clinical Oncology (ASCO) and serves on numerous breast cancer committees in other major oncology organizations. In addition, he serves as a consultant to the Oncology Drug Advisory Committee of the FDA.

"My belief," says Dr. Gradishar, "is that an educated patient will be a better advocate for her own health care."

Julie Gralow, M.D.

Julie Gralow , M.D., is Assistant Professor of Medical Oncology specializing in breast cancer at the University of Washington and the Fred Hutchinson Cancer Research Center. She is Director of the University of Washington's Women's Cancer Genetics and Risk Reduction Clinic and co-chairs the Southwest Oncology Group's Breast Cancer Center Committee. She is also Medical Director for Team Survivor Northwest, an exercise and fitness program for women cancer survivors. In that role, she has climbed mountains, participated in triathlons, biked in the 200-mile Seattle-to-Portland ride, rowed in a dragon boat, and had a great time while encouraging women cancer survivors to exercise and live healthy lives.

Generosa Grana, M.D., F.A.C.P

Dr. Grana is Associate Professor of Medicine at the Robert Wood Johnson Medical School in the division of Hematology and Oncology at the Cooper Hospital/University Medical Center in Camden, New Jersey. She is also Adjunct Assistant Professor at the Coriell Institute for Medical Research in Camden, New Jersey.

After graduating with a Bachelor of Science degree from the University of Notre Dame, Dr. Grana attended medical school at the Northwestern University School of Medicine in Chicago before doing her residency in internal medicine at Temple University in Philadelphia, Pennsylvania. Dr. Grana did her fellowship in hematology and oncology at the Fox Chase Cancer Center and Temple University in Philadelphia where she also did a post-doctoral fellowship in preventive oncology.

Dr. Grana is currently the Director of the Cancer Risk Evaluation Center as well as the Director of the Breast Cancer Program at the Cooper Hospital University Medical Center.

Dr. Grana has received numerous awards including the Johnson & Johnson Community Health Crystal Award in 1999, the American Cancer Society Silver Chalice Award in 1999 and the Best Doctors Award from the Philadelphia Magazine. She also serves on many committees including the vice chair of the Breast Health Task Force of the American Cancer Society New Jersey Division, and on the advisory groups for breast cancer and cancer prevention and control for the New Jersey State Commission on Cancer Research.

Dr. Grana has also made more than 32 national presentations, co-authored 13 publications, and presented 19 abstracts on breast cancer research.

Jennifer Griggs, M.D., M.P.H.

Jennifer Griggs, M.D., M.P.H., is a medical oncologist specializing in the treatment of breast cancer. She is Associate Professor, Department of Medicine in the Division of Hematology/Oncology at the University of Michigan in Ann Arbor. Dr. Griggs has received research funding from the National Institutes of Health, the Susan G. Komen Foundation, the Doris Duke Charitable Foundation, and the U.S. Department of Defense, and has written many articles and book chapters, including the oncology section of Cecil's Essentials of Medicine.

Jennifer has a special interest in cancer survivorship, patient-physician communication, and quality of care for women with breast cancer. She is particularly interested in the role of information support in quality of life. "Learning as much as possible about breast cancer helps a woman gain understanding and some control over a disease that too often has her feeling blown about like a leaf in the wind," she says. "And connecting to a community of breast cancer specialists and to other women with breast cancer immeasurably enhances a woman's circle of support. What I love about my work," she continues, "is the role I play in helping women make difficult decisions—especially with so much information for them to sort through—to find what's relevant, current, and reliable. Because of its unique format, breastcancer.org is poised to help women everywhere find the most dependable, up-to-the-minute information."

Dawn Hershman, M.D.

Dr. Dawn Hershman is Assistant Professor of Medicine at the Columbia University College of Physicians and Surgeons in the Division of Medical Oncology and has completed a Masters of Science in Biostatistics with an emphasis on patient-oriented research, at the Mailman School of Public Health.

She received her M.D. from The Albert Einstein College of Medicine, then trained in internal medicine at Columbia Presbyterian Medical Center where she served as Chief Resident, then completed a fellowship in Medical Oncology/Hematology. She is now the Director of the Clinical Breast Oncology Program. She has an interest and expertise in the area of health outcomes research with a specific interest in supportive care, racial disparities, and breast cancer survivorship.

Dr. Hershman has worked on several studies utilizing decision analysis models to determine the effectiveness of chemoprevention for groups of women at high risk of developing breast cancer. And she has published several papers from the linkage of the National Cancer Institute's Surveillance, Epidemiology and End-Result database with the Health Care Finance Administration's database, evaluating the utilization patterns of platinum-based chemotherapy in elderly patients with cancer.

She has several ongoing projects funded by the American Cancer Society evaluating the cognitive effects of chemotherapy. She has also been awarded grants from the American Society of Clinical Oncology and from The National Cancer Institute to support her investigation of bone loss patterns and osteoporosis prevention during treatment of breast cancer.

Carol Cherry, R.N., O.C.N., oncology nurse, Fox Chase Cancer Center, Pennsylvania

Marisa C. Weiss, M.D., breast radiation oncologist, Thomas Jefferson University Health System, Philadelphia, Pennsylvania

SOURCE: The American Cancer Society.

SOURCES: breastcancer.org. WebMD Medical Reference from the American College of Physicians: "Oncology: Breast Cancer." National Cancer Institute.

SOURCES: breastcancer.org. WebMD Medical Reference from the American College of Physicians: "Oncology: Breast Cancer." National Cancer Institutes.

ISBN: 978-1-4357-2137-1

Printed in the United Kingdom by
Lightning Source UK Ltd., Milton Keynes
139480UK00001B/33/P